# Medical Billing & Coding

## FOR

# DUMMIES®

## by Karen Smiley, CPC

WILEY

John Wiley & Sons, Inc.

**Medical Billing & Coding For Dummies®**

Published by
**John Wiley & Sons, Inc.**
111 River St.
Hoboken, NJ 07030-5774
www.wiley.com

Copyright © 2012 by John Wiley & Sons, Inc., Hoboken, New Jersey

Published by John Wiley & Sons, Inc., Hoboken, New Jersey

Published simultaneously in Canada

For general information on our other products and services, please contact our Customer Care Department within the U.S. at 877-762-2974, outside the U.S. at 317-572-3993, or fax 317-572-4002.

For technical support, please visit www.wiley.com/techsupport.

Wiley publishes in a variety of print and electronic formats and by print-on-demand. Some material included with standard print versions of this book may not be included in e-books or in print-on-demand. If this book refers to media such as a CD or DVD that is not included in the version you purchased, you may download this material at http://booksupport.wiley.com. For more information about Wiley products, visit www.wiley.com.

Library of Congress Control Number is available from the publisher.

ISBN 978-1-118-02172-9 (pbk); ISBN 978-1-118-22203-4 (ebk); ISBN 978-1-118-23614-7 (ebk); ISBN 978-1-118-26061-6 (ebk)

Manufactured in the United States of America

10 9 8 7 6 5 4 3 2 1

WILEY

# About the Author

**Karen Smiley** studied human anatomy in addition to Latin and Greek before settling down to raise a family. After several years working around the clock as a stay-at-home mom, she decided to enter the world of medical coding. After earning her certification, she found work at a nationally known practice management company and then found her way to employment at an Ambulatory Surgery Center. Along the way, she earned recognition at the local level and assisted in teaching coding — specifically cardio-vascular coding — to coding students. She recently joined a large billing company, where she uses her coding and billing skills to identify revenue cycle issues for various clients.

# Dedication

I dedicate this book to my family. Without their constant support and patience, completion of this book would not have been possible.

# Author's Acknowledgments

I wish to express my sincerest gratitude to Jen Dorsey. The technical component of this book is a compilation of my own knowledge and experience, but Jen sculpted the words into the final version that follows.

## Publisher's Acknowledgments

We're proud of this book; please send us your comments at http://dummies.custhelp.com. For other comments, please contact our Customer Care Department within the U.S. at 877-762-2974, outside the U.S. at 317-572-3993, or fax 317-572-4002.

Some of the people who helped bring this book to market include the following:

*Acquisitions, Editorial, and Vertical Websites*

**Editor:** Tracy L. Barr

**Executive Editor:** Lindsay Sandman Lefevere

**Assistant Editor:** David Lutton

**Editorial Program Coordinator:** Joe Niesen

**Technical Editor:** Barbara Fontaine

**Senior Editorial Manager:** Jennifer Ehrlich

**Editorial Manager:** Carmen Krikorian

**Editorial Assistant:** Rachelle S. Amick

**Art Coordinator:** Alicia B. South

**Cover Photos:** © iStockphoto.com / Helder Almeida

**Cartoons:** Rich Tennant (www.the 5thwave.com)

*Composition Services*

**Project Coordinator:** Sheree Montgomery

**Layout and Graphics:** Claudia Bell, Lavonne Roberts

**Proofreaders:** Melissa Cossell, ConText Editorial Services, Inc.

**Indexer:** Potomac Indexing, LLC

**Illustrator:** Kathryn Born

**Special Help:** Jennifer Dorsey

**Publishing and Editorial for Consumer Dummies**

    **Kathleen Nebenhaus,** Vice President and Executive Publisher

    **Kristin Ferguson-Wagstaffe,** Product Development Director

    **Ensley Eikenburg,** Associate Publisher, Travel

    **Kelly Regan,** Editorial Director, Travel

**Publishing for Technology Dummies**

    **Andy Cummings,** Vice President and Publisher

**Composition Services**

    **Debbie Stailey,** Director of Composition Services

# Contents at a Glance

# Table of Contents

# Introduction

$W$elcome to *Medical Billing & Coding For Dummies*! Consider this your personal guided tour to the profession that all physicians, hospitals, and clinics rely on to get paid in a timely fashion. This book shows you the ins and outs of the medical billing and coding profession, from the differences between the two jobs to how to prepare for and land a billing and coding job to what to expect after you're safely in that office chair.

As you read this book, you'll discover that medical billing and coding is a vital cog in the healthcare wheel. After all, the medical biller and coder is the rainmaker of the healthcare industry, turning the healthcare provider's documentation into payment.

Medical billing and coding is way more than codes and insider jargon, though. It's also about working with people and knowing how to interact with each type of person or business you come in contact with, from patients and physicians to fellow coders and insurance reps — a virtual who's who of the medical world — and you'll be right in the middle of them all!

## About This Book

The world of medical billing and coding, what with all the terminology you must master and the codes you need to know, can seem big and a bit daunting at times. After all, there's a lot to remember and so, so many codes. But don't worry: Parsing the ins and outs of all the details on how to enter the correct code is what those super-technical coding books are for. Think of *this* book as a friendly guide to all the twists and turns you'll encounter in your medical billing and coding world, from taking the certification exam and finding a job to working with insurance companies and deciphering physician documentation.

Not only do I share the ins and outs of the profession itself and what to expect on the job, but I also tell you what you need to know to succeed.

What this book isn't is a book of codes. Tons of great resources are out there that list all the codes you need to do your job properly, and I recommend that you have them handy. Instead, this book is a friendly take on the job as a whole. My main goal is to introduce you to the wider world of medical billing and coding so that you are prepped and ready to scrub in for this challenging, evolving, and always exciting career.

# Conventions Used in This Book

Think of this book as a grand tour into the world of medical billing and coding. To help you navigate through all the wonderful information here, I've used the following conventions:

- ✔ **Bulleted lists:** What can I say? I'm a list person. In these lists, you'll find key points in a quick, easy-to-read fashion.

- ✔ *Italics:* I use *italic* to highlight new words or terms that you may not be familiar with and that merit a quick definition. I also use italics if I want to emphasize something.

- ✔ **Boldfaced:** I use boldface for the action part of numbered steps and to highlight key concepts and phrases in bulleted lists.

- ✔ `Monofont`: I use this font for web addresses.

# What You're Not to Read

Medical billing and coding is a pretty big field, and I cover all the basics in this book. But just because there's a lot to say doesn't mean you have to read everything that's in here. I included some stuff just because it's interesting or provides background details that you may find helpful. So that you can easily distinguish between the need-to-know stuff and the stuff you can safely pass by without impeding your understanding of medical billing and coding, I note the info you can skip:

- ✔ **Text in sidebars:** The sidebars are the shaded boxes that appear here and there. You may find the info in these boxes interesting or fun, but it's not necessary reading.

- ✔ **Anything with a Technical Stuff icon attached:** This information is interesting but not critical to your understanding of medical billing and coding.

Of course, you can also skip whatever else you don't want to read. After all, I organized and wrote this book so that you can easily find the topics that interest you.

# Foolish Assumptions

In writing this book, I made some assumptions about you:

- ✔ You're a medically minded individual who is interested in pursuing a career in medical billing and coding and has no previous coding experience.
- ✔ You're a current medical professional who is looking to switch to the coding side of the industry.
- ✔ You're a medical billing and coding student who is looking for information on certifications, job hunting, and the career in general.

Regardless of why you picked up this book, you can find the info you need to pursue your medical billing and coding career goals with confidence.

# How This Book Is Organized

We don't mess around with much extraneous info here in *For Dummies* land. You want to know the most important info in a quick, easy-to-read manner, and I want to give it to you. To that end, I divided the topic into parts. In each part are chapters, each of which focuses on a particular aspect of billing and coding.

## Part 1: Getting to Know Medical Billing and Coding

This part helps you start your journey. Here you can find an introduction to medical billing and coding, information on what differentiates a medical coder from a medical biller, and how the two function together. I also explain what job options are available to you in the medical billing and coding profession, from working for in an office or hospital to freelancing from home.

# Part II: Boning Up on the Need-to-Knows of Your Profession

In this part, I tell you all about the most vital tidbits you need to know to succeed in the medical billing and coding profession. Here you can find information on compliance (basically the rules and laws you need to follow), medical terminology (the language used in medical documentation), and medical necessity (the idea that, if a service is to be reimbursed, it must be medically necessary). I wrap up this part by introducing you to the payers: the commercial insurance companies and federal insurance programs (Medicare and others) you'll deal with daily.

# Part III: Keys to Becoming a Professional: Getting Certified

In this part, I lay out the ground work that can help you score that medical billing and coding job. Here you discover what certification is, how to go about getting the certification you want, and how to find a training program that prepares you for the certification exam and your career.

Finally, just in case you want to gild the lily a bit, I tell you how to add some specialty certifications and participate in continuing ed programs to your already sparkling credentials.

# Part IV: Dealing with the Nitty-Gritty On-the-Job Details

Say you get that dream job — and you will! Now's the time to delve into the nitty-gritty details of the life of a medical biller/coder. In this part, I walk you through the claim-filing process and explain how to resolve disputes and appeal claims that get denied.

# Part V: Working with Stakeholders

I can't stress this enough: Medical billing and coding is, in the end, all about people. Yes, it's true that you'll spend a great deal of time working with codes and software and what seems to be an endless parade of compliance rules and regulations. But it's also true that people are both your clients and your payers, so knowing how to interface with them is important. In this part, I introduce you to your stakeholders, the people and organizations that depend on your coding.

## Part VI: The Part of Tens

Ah, the good old Part of Tens. Who doesn't love a list? Here you can find three useful lists to help you navigate the exciting world of medical billing and coding. I tell you how to avoid common billing and coding problems and what acronyms you'll encounter on a daily basis. I also share with you some of the best tips and pointers from medical billing and coding professionals.

# Icons Used in This Book

As you read this book, you'll notice icons peppered throughout the text. Consider these signposts directing you to special kinds of information. Here's what each icon means:

This icon marks tips and tricks you can use to help you succeed in the day-to-day tasks of medical billing and coding.

This icon highlights passages that are good to keep in mind as you master the medical billing and coding profession.

This icon alerts you to common mistakes that can trip you up when you are coding or following up on a denial.

This icon indicates something cool and perhaps a little offbeat from the discussion at hand. Feel free to skip these bits.

# *Where to Go from Here*

This book is designed to be easy to navigate and easy to read, no matter what topic you're interested in. Looking for information on certification exams? Head to Chapter 7. Want to know how to file an appeal? Chapter 14 has the information you need.

Of course, if you feel confident that you already know the basics on medical billing and coding and you want to dive into the middle of this book, feel free. That said, getting a strong idea of what the medical billing and coding job entails can be incredibly useful if you're a bit on the fence about whether this is the job for you. If that description fits you, start in Part I, where you can find some really useful overview-type info.

Bottom line: Go wherever you want. After all, it's your life, it's your future, and this profession is yours for the taking. Go for it!

# Part I

# Getting to Know Medical Billing and Coding

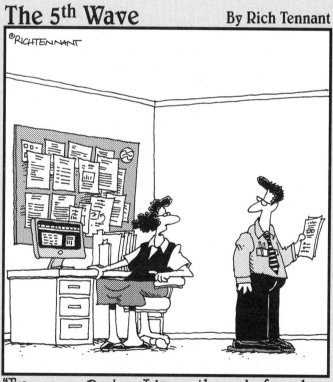

The 5th Wave          By Rich Tennant

"Excuse me, Doctor. I know the code for when you're late because of a golf game, but what's the billing code for whatever it is that you do here?"

## In this part . . .

Time to meet your new profession: medical billing and coding. This part fills you in on the who, what, when, where, and why of the profession known as the lifeline of the medical industry. As a medical biller and coder, you're the connection between providers and the people who pay them.

These chapters fill you in on all the general details about working in the medical industry as a biller and coder, from the basics of the job to what job options are available to you.

# Chapter 1

# Dipping Your Toes in Medical Billing and Coding

*In This Chapter*

▶ Getting to know the industry

▶ Deciding whether the job is right for you

▶ Choosing a certification

▶ Planning your education

*W*elcome to the world of medical billing and coding! No other job in the medical field affects more lives than this one because everyone involved in the healthcare experience, from the patient and front office staff to providers and payers, relies on you. You are, so to speak, the touchstone in the medical industry.

A lot rests on your shoulders as the biller and coder. With this responsibility comes great power, and that power must be treated with respect and integrity. In this chapter, I take you on a very brief tour of what medical billing and coding entails. I hope you find, as I have, that working as a medical biller/coder is a challenging and rewarding job that takes you right into the heart of the medical industry.

# Coding versus Billing: They Really Are Two Jobs

Although many people refer to billing and coding as if it were one job function (a convention I use in this book unless I'm referring to specific functions), billing and coding really are two distinct careers. In the following sections, I briefly describe the tasks and functions associated with each job and give you some things to think about to determine which path you want to pursue:

- ✔ The medical coder deciphers the documentation of a patient's interaction with a healthcare provider (physician, surgeon, nursing staff, and so on) and determines the appropriate procedure (CPT) and diagnosis code(s) to reflect the services provided.

- ✔ The biller then takes the assigned codes and any required insurance information, enters them into the billing software, and then submits the claim to the payer (often an insurance company) to be paid. The biller also follows up on the claim as necessary.

- ✔ Both medical billers and coders are responsible for a variety of tasks, and they're in constant interaction with a variety of people (you can read about the various stakeholders in Part V). Consider these examples:

  - • Because they're responsible for billing insurance companies and patients correctly, medical billers have daily interaction with both patients and insurance companies to ensure that claims are paid in a reasonable time.

  - • To ensure coding accuracy, coders often find themselves querying physicians regarding any questions they may have about the procedures that were performed during the patient encounter and educating other office staff on gathering required information.

  - • Billers (but sometimes coders, too) have the responsibility for explaining charges to patients, particularly when patients need help understanding their payment obligations, such as co-insurance and copayments, that their insurance policies specify.

- ✔ When submitting claims to the insurance company, billers are responsible for verifying the correct billing format, assigning the proper modifier(s), and submitting all required documentation with each claim.

In short, medical billers and coders together collect information and documentation, code claims accurately so that physicians get paid in a timely manner, and follow up with payers to make sure that the money finds its way to the client's bank account. Both jobs are crucial to the office cash flow of any healthcare provider, and they may be done by two separate people or by one individual, depending upon the size of the office.

For the complete lowdown on exactly what billers and coders do, check out Chapter 2 for general information and Part IV, which provides detailed information on claims processing.

# A Day in the Life of a Claim

When you're not interfacing with the three Ps — patients, providers, and payers — you'll be doing the "meat and potatoes" work of your day: coding claims to convert physician- or specialist-performed services into revenue.

*Claims processing* refers to the overall work of submitting and following up on claims. Here in a nutshell is the general process of claims submission, which begins almost as soon as the patient enters the provider's office:

1. **The patient hands over her insurance card and fills out a demographic form at the time of arrival.**

   The demographic form includes info such as patient name, date of birth, address, Social Security or driver's license number, the name of the policyholder, and any additional information about the policyholder if the policyholder is someone other than the patient. At this time, patient also presents a government-issued photo ID so that you can verify that she is actually the insured member.

   Using someone else's insurance coverage is fraud. So is submitting a claim that misrepresents an encounter. All providers are responsible for verifying patient identity, and they can be held liable for fraud committed in their office.

2. **After the initial paperwork is complete, the patient encounter with the service provider or physician occurs, followed by the provider documenting the billable services.**

3. **The coder abstracts the billable codes, based on the physician documentation.**

4. **The coding goes to the biller who enters the information into the appropriate claim form in the billing software.**

   After the biller enters the coding information into the software, the software sends the claim either directly to the payer or to a clearinghouse, which sends the claim to the appropriate payer for reimbursement.

If everything goes according to plan, and all the moving parts of the billing and coding process work as they should, your claim gets paid, and no follow up is necessary. For a detailed discussion of the claims process from beginning to end, check out Chapters 11, 12, and 13).

Of course, things may not go as planned, and the claim will get hung up somewhere — often for missing or incomplete information — or it may be denied. If either of these happen, you must follow up to discover the problem and then resolve it. Chapter 14 has all the details you need about this part of your job.

# Keeping Abreast of What Every Biller/Coder Needs to Know

If you're going to work in the medical billing and coding industry (and you will!), you must familiarize yourself with three big "must-know" items: compliance (following the regulations established by the United States Office of Inspector General, or OIG), medical terminology (the language healthcare providers use to describe the diagnosis and treatment they provide), and medical necessity (the diagnosis that makes the provided service necessary). In the following sections, I introduce you to these concepts. For more info, head to Part II.

## Complying with OIG regulations

In the United States, as in many countries, healthcare is a regulated industry, and you have to follow certain regulations. In the U.S. these rules are established by the Office of Inspector General. The regulations are designed to prevent fraud and abuse by healthcare providers, and as a medical biller or coder, you must familiarize yourself with the basics of compliance.

Being *in compliance* basically means an office or individual has established a program to run the practice under the regulations as set forth by the U.S. Office of Inspector General (OIG).

You can thank something called HIPAA for setting the bar for compliance. The standard of securing the confidentiality of healthcare information was established by the enactment of the Health Insurance Portability and Accountability Act (HIPAA). This legislation guarantees certain rights to individuals with regard to their healthcare. Check out Chapter 4 for more info on compliance, HIPAA, and the OIG.

## Learning the lingo: Medical terminology

Everyone knows that doctors speak a different language. Turns out that that language is often Latin or Greek. By putting together a variety of Latin and Greek prefixes and suffixes, physicians and other healthcare providers can describe any number of illnesses, injuries, conditions, and procedures.

As a coder, you need to become familiar with these prefixes and suffixes so that you can figure out precisely what procedure codes to use. By mastering the meaning of each segment of a medical term, you'll be able to quickly make sense of the terminology that you use every day.

You can read about the most common prefixes and suffixes in Chapter 5.

## Proving medical necessity

Before a payer (such as an insurance company) will reimburse the provider, the provider must show that rendering the services was necessary. Setting a broken leg is necessary, for example, only when the leg is broken. Similarly, prenatal treatment and newborn delivery is necessary only when the patient is pregnant.

To prove medical necessity, the coder must make sure that the diagnosis code supports the treatment given. Therefore, you must be familiar with diagnosis codes and their relationship to the procedure codes. You can find out more about medical necessity in Chapter 5.

Insurance companies are usually the parties responsible for paying the doctor or other medical provider for services rendered. However, they pay only for procedures that are medically necessary to the well-being of the patient, their client. Each procedure billed must be linked to a diagnosis that supports the medical necessity for the procedure. All diagnosis and procedures are worded in medical terminology.

# Deciding Which Job Is Right for You

If you think the idea of working with everyone from patients to payers sounds good and working a claim through the coding process seems right up your alley, then you can start to think about which particular jobs in the field might be a good fit for you. Luckily, you have lots of options. You just need to know where to look and what kind of job is right for you. I give you some things to think about in the following sections.

## Going through your workplace options

Before you crack open the classifieds, give some thought to what sort of environment you want to work in. You can find billing and coding work in all sorts of places, such as

- Physician offices
- Hospitals
- Nursing homes
- Outpatient facilities
- Billing companies
- Home healthcare services
- Durable medical good providers
- Practice management companies
- Federal government agencies
- Commercial payers

Which type of facility you choose depends on the kind of environment that fits your personality. For example, you may want to work in the fast-paced, volume-heavy work that's common in a hospital. Or maybe the controlled chaos of a smaller physician's office is more up your alley.

Other considerations for choosing a particular area is what you can gain from working there. A larger office or a hospital setting is great for new coders because you get to work under the direct supervision of a more experienced coding staff. A billing company that specializes in specific provider types lets you become an expert in a particular are. In many physician offices, you get to develop a broader expertise because you're not only in charge of coding, but you're also responsible for following up on accounts receivable and chasing submitted claims.

To find out more about your workplace options and the advantages and disadvantages that come with each, head to Chapter 3.

## *Thinking about your dream job*

Although you can't predict the future, you can begin to put some thought into your long-term career goals and how you can reach them. Here are some factors to consider when thinking about what kind of billing/coding job you want:

- **The kind of job you want to do and the tasks you want to spend your time performing:** Refer to the earlier sections "A Day in the Life of a Claim" and "Keeping Abreast of What Every Biller/Coder Needs to Know" for more on the job-related tasks. Chapter 2 has a complete discussion of billing and coding job functions.

✔ **Where you plan to seek employment and in what kind of setting:**
The preceding section gives you a quick idea of what your options are.
Chapter 3 gives you more detail.

✔ **The type of certification potential employers prefer and the time commitment involved:** Many billing or practice management companies, for
example, are contractually obligated to their clients to employ only certified medical coders to perform the coding.

✔ **The type of training program(s) available in your area:** Many reputable training programs are associated with the two main biller/coder
credentialing organizations, the AAPC (formerly the American Academy
of Professional Coders) and AHIMA (American Health Information
Management Association), each of which tends to focus on a particular
area: AAPC certification is generally associated with coding in physicians' offices; AHIMA certification is generally associated with hospital
coding. For information about finding a training program and your
options, head to Chapter 8.

Take a few minutes (or hours!) now to think over these points. Trust me: It's
time well spent before you jump on the billing and coding bandwagon.

# Prepping for Your Career: Training Programs and Certifications

Breaking into the billing and coding industry takes more than a wink and
a smile (though I'm sure yours are lovely). It takes training from reputable
institutions and certification from a reputable credentialing organization. The
next sections have the details.

## An overview of your certification options

To score a job as a biller and coder, you must get certified by a reputable credentialing organization such as the American Health Information
Management Association (AHIMA) or the AAPC (formerly known as the
American Academy of Professional Coders). In Chapter 7, I tell you everything you need to know about these organization. Here's a quick overview:

✔ The AAPC is the credentialing organization that offers Certified
Professional Coder (CPC) credentials. The AAPC training focuses on
physician offices and outpatient hospital-based coding.

✔ The AHIMA coding certifications — Correct Coding Specialist (CCS) and Certified Coding Associate (CCA) — are intended to certify the coder who has demonstrated proficiency in inpatient and outpatient hospital-based coding, while the Correct Coding Specialist Physician-Based (CCS-P) is, as its name indicates, for coders who work for individual physicians.

All sorts of other specialty certifications are also available, which you can read more about in Chapter 10.

To choose which certification — AHIMA or AAPC — best fits your career goals, first think about the type of training program you want. Second, examine your long-term career goals. What kind of medical billing and coding job do you ultimately want to do, in what sort of facility do you want to work, and how do you want to spend your time each day?

To get certified, you must pass an exam administered by the credentialing organization. Head to Chapter 9 for exam details and info on how to sign up for one.

## Going back to school

Sharpen your pencils, get a sweet new backpack, and shine up an apple for the teacher because you're going back to school. That's right, school. It's your first stop on the way to Medical Billing and Coding Land. The good news is that medical coding is one of the few medical careers with fewer education requirements. Translation: You won't be spending decades preparing for your new career. Most billing and coding programs get you up and running in a relatively short amount of time, often less than two years.

After you successfully complete a training program, you receive a *certificate of completion*. Note that this is different from achieving *certification*. To get your certification, you still have to take certification exams offered by the credentialing bodies after graduation. Fortunately, a solid medical coding and billing program provides you with the knowledge necessary to ace the exams and gain entry-level certification. Most programs offer training in the following:

✔ Human anatomy and physiology

✔ Medical terminology

✔ Medical documentation

✔ Medical coding, including proper use of modifiers

✔ Medical billing

✔ Claims filing

✔ Medical insurance, including commercial payers and government programs

You can read all about your educational options — from abbreviated study programs to more inclusive extended programs — in Chapter 8, where I highlight the advantages of some programs and the pitfalls of others.

# Planning for the Future

As soon as you get your first billing and coding job — and probably even before that — you'll start hearing about something called ICD-10, which is the 10th edition of the International Classification of Diseases (hence, the ICD), the common system of codes that classifies every disease or health problem you code. These diagnosis codes represent a generalized description of the disease or injury that was the catalyst for the patient/physician encounter. As a biller/coder, you use the ICD every day.

ICD codes are also used to classify diseases and other health problems that are recorded on many types of health records, including death certificates, to help provide national mortality and morbidity rates. The ninth edition of the ICD classification (ICD-9) has been used in the United States since 1979. But ICD-10 is coming, ready or not, and it isn't just an update to the old version. ICD-10 is a completely new edition, with all codes rearranged and placed in different areas.

ICD-9 is the old-school coding classification system, while ICD-10 is the new kid in town, and the differences between the two are fairly significant. For starters, ICD-9 has just over 14,000 diagnosis codes and almost 4,000 procedural codes. In contrast, ICD-10 contains more than 68,000 diagnosis codes (clinical modification codes) and more than 72,000 procedural codes. Other differences involve how the codes are presented (the number of characters, for example) and how you interpret them (deciphering the characters to know what particular groupings mean).

As of this writing, all healthcare providers are obligated to be ICD-10–ready by October 1, 2014. Because getting everyone the world over on the same page, so to speak, is such a gargantuan job, ICD-10 is being implemented in phases for just about anyone who has anything to do with using it.

The World Health Organization (WHO) uses the data gleaned from your coding to analyze the health of large population groups and monitor diseases and other health problems for all members of the global community. For your purposes, you can think of the ICD codes as the language you speak when coding so that organizations like WHO can do the work of keeping the world healthy.

Changing over to ICD-10 could do you good. Currently, medical billing and coding jobs comprise one-fifth of the healthcare workforce, a number that is expected to grow. Transitioning to ICD-10 is expected to increase the demand for medical coders because it will make the coding and billing process more complicated and time-consuming. You can read more about ICD-10 in Chapter 15.

# Chapter 2

# Exploring the Billing and Coding Professions

*M*edical billing and coding specialists are the healthcare professionals responsible for converting patient data from treatment records and insurance information into revenue. They take all those complicated codes and turn them into language the insurance companies and other payers can understand. The healthcare industry depends on qualified medical billers and skilled medical coders to accurately record, register, and keep track of each patient's account so that the docs get paid and the patients get charged only for services they receive.

Although they're frequently clumped together, medical billing and medical coding are actually two distinct jobs. In this chapter, I discuss each separately.

*Note:* In this chapter, I offer a very brief overview of the tasks that billers and coders perform. For a detailed discussion of the billing and coding process, head to Part IV.

## The Lowdown on Medical Coding

The coder's job is to extract the appropriate billable services from the documentation that has been provided. The coder is given the office notes and/or the operative report as dictated by the physician. From this documentation, the coder identifies any and all billable procedures and assigns the correct diagnosis and procedure codes. The coder also identifies whether a procedure that is often included with another procedure should be billed on its own (or, in coder-speak, *unbundled*) to allow for additional reimbursement. (To be eligible for unbundling, the documentation must indicate that extra time and effort was required or that a procedure that is normally included in the primary procedure was done at a separate site or time and was necessary to ensure a positive outcome for the patient.)

That's the nuts-and-bolts stuff. To do the job of medical coder well, however, you must be aware that medical coding requires a daily commitment to remaining ethical despite pressures from employers who are looking at the bottom line and don't understand the laws and procedural mandates a coder must follow. I have heard physicians tell coders to just use the code with the highest revenue potential. This philosophy may be what is best in the short term for the provider's bottom line, but when an auditor comes around to investigate, that money is going back with interest. So the first order every day for the coder is to be mindful of her ethical duty to the profession, physicians, and patients.

The key to optimal reimbursement is full documentation by the provider (the physician, for example, who sees the patient and performs the procedure) coupled with full *extraction,* or identification, of billable procedures by the coder. Everyone — from the doc to you, the coder — has to dot every *i* and cross every *t*.

In the following sections, I take you through the different tasks you'll perform as you prepare claims for reimbursement.

## Verifying documentation

As noted earlier, the job of coder starts with the documentation provided by the physician. This documentation can take the form of an operative report or an office note.

Physicians are trained to document their work, so consider them partners in the coding enterprise. They (or a member of their staff) note all the information needed to treat a particular patient before the paperwork hits the coder's desk.

### Checking operative reports

An *operative report* is the document that is transcribed from the physician's dictation of the patient encounter. It describes in detail exactly what was done during the surgery. Operative reports are normally set into a template, which serves as an outline that identifies the reason for the procedure, what illness or injury was confirmed during the procedure, and finally the procedure(s) that were performed.

The basic format of an operative report includes the following:

✔ Patient name and date of birth

✔ Operating physician

✔ Date of service

✔ Preoperative diagnosis (the diagnosis based the examination and preoperative testing)

✔ Postoperative diagnosis (the diagnosis based on what the doctor found during the surgery)

✔ Procedure(s) performed (an outline of the procedures done)

✔ Body of the operative report (a description of everything that was stated in the postoperative diagnosis and procedure performed sections)

Put simply, verifying documentation is a fact-checking gig. Here's what you need to check:

✔ That procedures stated as performed in the heading of the operative report are substantiated in the body of the report.

✔ The diagnosis provides medical necessity for the procedure and that the procedure(s) listed in the outline are documented in the body of the operative report. *Medical necessity* is simply the reason for the visit or surgery; it defines the disease process or injury (head to Chapter 5 for details). Before payers reimburse the provider, they have to know why the visit was necessary.

As a coder, you rely on the information in the body of the operative report to verify the documentation. If the body doesn't support the rest of the operative report (the operative report doesn't mention a procedure listed in the procedures performed section, for example, or the description isn't detailed enough), then you're responsible for asking the surgeon to clarify. Remember: If the doctor doesn't say it in the operative report, regardless of how obvious it seems, *it was not done.*

### Checking office notes

All physician services are coded and billed based upon physician documentation. When coding office procedures or verifying the level of evaluation and management code that is appropriate for the visit, you rely on the physician's office notes. An office note typically documents the patient's symptoms, the physician's findings, and the plan for treatment, including a follow-up plan.

If you believe that a higher level of service was performed, asking a physician for clarification is certainly acceptable, but coding a procedure that's not documented is not acceptable. Coding is not a job for those who like to second-guess. You can't assume you know what the doctor meant or intended and code based on your assumptions. Therefore, make sure you add "clarifying information" to your list of daily jobs as a coder.

---

# It's a bird! It's a plane! It's Super-bill!

A super-bill is a form created specifically for an individual office or provider. It normally is prepopulated with the patient's information, including insurance copay, and contains the most common diagnosis and procedural codes used by the office. It may also have a section that indicates the need for follow-up appointments and should also have a space for the physician's signature.

The super-bill is a great tool for the provider for billing purposes and also proves helpful for keeping track of each patient's visits. In many offices, the super-bill has been replaced by the electronic health record (EHR), an all-electronic method of patient recordkeeping.

Super-bills, wonderful as they are, can also be the bane of the coder's existence. Although checking off billable procedures is certainly easier for the provider, they may overlook adding the detail necessary to support the procedures (and level of the visit) indicated on the bill. If the chart doesn't match the super-bill, it's back to square one for the coder.

---

## Following up on unclear documentation

As I explain in the preceding sections, the physician documents all procedures he performs. If he doesn't state a procedure in his dictation (in his operative report) or note it in the physician's notes, regardless of how obvious it may seem, *it was not done.*

 The chant of the medical coder always comes in handy. When in doubt or faced with incomplete documentation, remember: "If the doctor didn't say it, it wasn't done." Period.

When the documentation is missing or ambiguous, it's your responsibility to clarify with the physician. Although some physicians become defensive or irritated when the coder questions the documentation, those who understand that your questions can maximize their reimbursement will gladly amend the documentation to clear up the problem.

## Assigning diagnosis and procedure codes

Time to play "Name that Illness!" Upon reading the operative report or office notes, you must identify the illness or disease and find the corresponding diagnosis code in the International Classification of Diseases (ICD) book, Volumes 1 and 2. (The current edition is ICD-9, but it will soon be ICD-10; you can read about the transition in Chapter 15.) This book is the bible of coding, containing all the diagnosis codes.

After finding the diagnosis codes, you then look up the procedure codes that best describe the work done, using one of the following books:

- ✔ **The Current Procedural Terminology (CPT) book:** The CPT book contains all the procedure codes as determined by the American Medical Association (AMA) and includes the definition of each procedure. Physicians and outpatient facilities choose a code from the CPT book.

- ✔ **The ICD-9 Volume 3 book:** Hospital inpatient procedures are chosen from the ICD-9 Volume 3 book.

Because so many different codes and corresponding procedures exist, you may suffer from "coding drama." Coding a procedure with a lot of moving parts can get a bit complicated. Sure, capturing all the procedures that were performed during a surgery is important, for example, but they each must be separately billable or have involved extra work by the surgeon in order to justify unbundling them (or billing them separately). The point? Coding can get pretty complicated. Before you panic, keep this in mind: Coding a procedure is simple if you remember to break it down into small bites.

### Physician coding

Physician coding is just what it sounds like: coding diagnoses and procedures representing the work performed by a physician. Under certain circumstances, work performed in an outpatient setting, such as an ambulatory surgery center (ASC), also uses physician coding.

Physician offices, ambulatory surgery centers, and other outpatient facilities use the CPT code sets to represent the procedure performed. Physician claims are submitted on the HCFA/CMS-1500 claim form. In most circumstances, facilities bill commercial carriers on the UB-04 claim form. Both of these forms are discussed later in this chapter.

### Facility coding

Coding for facility reimbursement often pertains to hospital coding. Specific coding and billing guidelines exist for hospital billing. If you are working as a facility coder in a hospital, you use Volume 3 of the ICD-9 book to identify the procedures.

Basically, facility coding is for the hospital inpatient setting. Outpatient centers, including those run by the hospital, use physician coding.

## Transforming visits into revenue

After the procedure codes and diagnosis codes are entered into the office billing software, the billing process officially begins.

In many offices, the claim is out of the coder's hands at this point because the actual billing part of the process falls to the medical biller who takes the coding information and submits it for payment (you can read about that job in the next section). Nevertheless, the claim may return in the form of a denial from the payer.

Often, if a claim is denied for medical necessity (refer to Chapter 5), it is returned to coding for clarification or verification so that it can be resubmitted.

## Determining whether medical coding is for you

As you decide whether medical coding is a job you'd like and do well at, consider these points:

- As a medical coder, you're responsible for extracting the correct procedure code from the physician's documentation. To do this task well, you must have a strong command of the language, be a good reader, and be very detail oriented.

  In fact, the job of coder is especially attractive to those who are skilled at analyzing data. Every procedure performed in a medical setting has a specific code assigned to it, and it needs to be coded properly to ensure correct billing and maximum reimbursement for the physician or facility.

- You're responsible for recognizing when information is unclear or missing from the documentation and for clarifying with the physician any ambiguous wording in the documentation.

- You must stay current on correct coding guidelines and the ever-changing procedure codes as determined by the American Medical Association and the Centers for Medicare & Medicaid Services.

  Check out www.ama-assn.org and www.cms.gov for the most up-to-date coding changes.

- As a coder, you may not have much interaction with insurance companies and patients because they tend to spend most of their time in the office working on claims. So if you think coding is the job for you, know that you'll have more face time with your computer than with patients.

# On the Job with the Medical Biller

After the coder does her thing, it's time for the medical biller to step up to the plate. As the biller, you're responsible for billing insurance companies and patients.

When you submit claims to the insurance company, you're responsible for verifying the correct billing format, assigning the proper modifier(s), and submitting all required documentation with each claim. In most offices, claims are submitted through billing software. Learning to use the software is essential to successful billing and will be a major part of your on-the-job training after you're hired. In the following sections, I highlight the key parts of your job as a medical biller.

A claim that has been well documented and correctly coded and billed should generate a timely payment for the physician, which is the goal of both the medical coder and biller.

## Knowing the payers and staying abreast of their idiosyncrasies

Most providers have contracts with multiple commercial payers (basically insurance companies), as well as government payers, such as Medicare. Here's a very brief overview of the kinds of payers and organizations you'll work with as a medical biller:

- ✔ **Commercial insurance:** These are private insurance carriers, and they fall into a variety of categories, each of which has particular rules regarding what's covered, when, and how providers get reimbursed. Preferred provider plans (PPOs), health maintenance plans (HMOs), and point of service plans (POSs) are just a few you'll deal with.

- ✔ **Networks:** Some commercial payers and providers participate in networks. A *network* is essentially a middle man who functions as an agent for commercial payers by pricing claims (that is, setting the fees associated with medical procedures) for them.

- ✔ **Third-party administrators:** These intermediaries either operate as a network or access networks to price claims, and they often handle claims processing for employers who self-insure their employees rather than use a traditional group health plan.

- ✔ **Government payers:** These include governmental insurance programs that offer benefits to particular groups. Examples of government payers include Medicare (the elderly and qualifying disabled people), Medicaid (the poor), Tricare (military members and their families), and so on.

Chapter 6 goes into a great deal of detail on all the things you need to know about these payers. What you need to know now is that each has its own rules and guidelines that must be followed to secure reimbursement. As a medical biller, you must be familiar with the eccentricities of each payer. You never know what you might need to know about a payer, such as which modifiers are accepted, how the payer views bilateral procedures, and what kind of documentation the payer requires. Most Workers' Compensation carriers, for example, require that procedural notes be included with *all* claims, even if doing so means they get the same operative report from the facility and the surgeon.

Taking the time upfront to learn what each payer requires can save you a lot of time when you're in the groove of billing. Who wants to get tripped up by not knowing a payer's documentation needs? Not you, rock star. So bone up on this information early and then hit your mental "refresh" button often by staying abreast of the latest payer information. You can read about the different payers in Chapter 6.

## *Paper or plastic? Billing each payer correctly*

As with just about everything else in life, billing and coding is going paperless. Remember those giant sliding file cabinets in the doctor's office? They're either gone or are being used to store the office holiday decorations. The Health Insurance Portability and Accountability Act (HIPAA) now makes it necessary to bill most claims electronically.

Most payers accept electronic claims, although some still require paper claims. It's your responsibility to know which method will be accepted. This information is contained in the payer contract, but sometimes you need to call and ask how to submit the claim.

You'll encounter various formats or platforms of electronic claim submissions. For that reason, as the biller, you also need to make sure that the correct format is linked to each individual payer. Fortunately, this information isn't too difficult to find: The patient's insurance card normally has claim submission information on it, and of course, you can always call the payer to check prior to submitting a claim if you have any uncertainty.

For several decades, medical billing was entirely on paper. Then medical practice management software was developed and made claim processing more efficient. Although paper claims may soon be extinct due to the introduction of the HIPAA (covered in Chapter 4), certain payers are exempt and will continue to accept and possibly require paper claims.

In the following sections, I introduce you to the forms you'll encounter as a medical biller.

### The CMS-1500 form

The Centers for Medicare & Medicaid 1500 (CMS-1500) form, formerly known as a Health Care Financing Administration-1500 (HCFA-1500) form, is the paper form used to submit claims for professional services (see Figure 2-1). Physicians and clinical practitioners submit their claims on this form, which is printed in red ink and contains spaces for all the necessary information. Directions for completing the form are printed on the back of each one.

Various forms have been used in the past, and it's essential that you use the current, or correct edition, when submitting claim via a paper form.

The HCFA/CMS-1500 form is split into three sections. Section one is patient information. All this information should be in the patient's registration form. Section two is for procedural and diagnostic information, which should be on the super-bill or coding form. Section three is for the provider information. See? Easy as 1-2-3.

### The UB-04/CMS-1450 form

The Uniform Bill 04 (UB-04) claim form, also called the CMS-1450 or just plain UB in some circles, is used by facilities for their health insurance billing. Hospitals, rehabilitation centers, ambulatory surgery centers, and clinics must bill their services on the UB-04 form in order to get paid by commercial payers. There are 84 boxes on the UB-04. Required fields on the UB include revenue codes, bill type, and sometimes value codes in addition to the information required in the HCFA. Just as with the HCF/CMS-1500, the directions are printed on the back of the form.

## Checking the claim over prior to submission

As I mention previously, as a biller, you'll receive the claim form from the coder and then prepare it for submission. In addition to knowing which submittal method to use — paper or electronic — you also need to check the claim over to make sure all the necessary information is included. This is one of the reasons why, even though you're not a coder, you need to understand the medical codes used.

In addition, you also need to know how to use modifiers correctly. The coder may be responsible for assigning modifiers based on correct coding edits, but the biller is ultimately responsible for making sure that payer-specific (or provider-specific) modifiers are on the claim prior to submission. For information on modifiers and checking the claim over before submitting, head to Chapter 12.

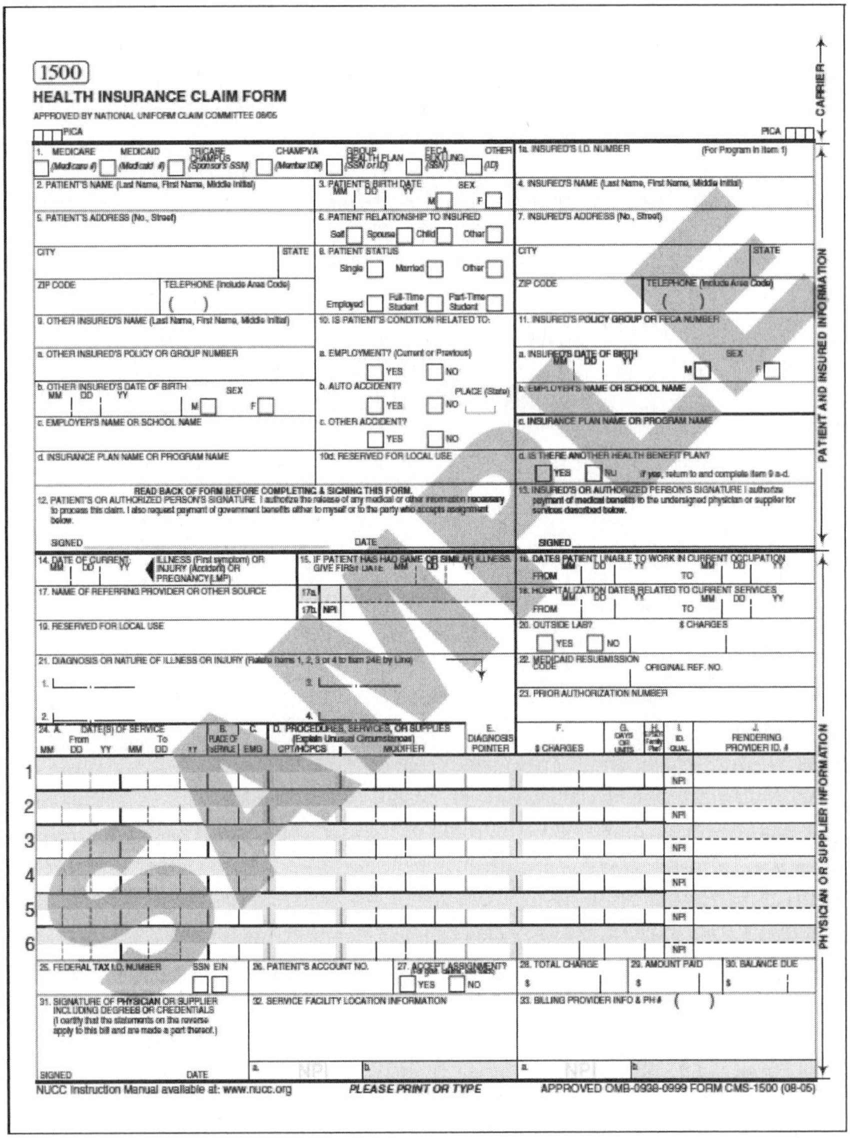
1500
HEALTH INSURANCE CLAIM FORM
APPROVED BY NATIONAL UNIFORM CLAIM COMMITTEE 08/05
PICA
1. MEDICARE MEDICAID TRICARE CHAMPUS CHAMPVA GROUP HEALTH PLAN FECA BLK LUNG OTHER
(Medicare #) (Medicaid #) (Sponsor's SSN) (Member ID#) (SSN or ID) (SSN) (ID)
1a. INSURED'S I.D. NUMBER (For Program in Item 1)
2. PATIENT'S NAME (Last Name, First Name, Middle Initial)
3. PATIENT'S BIRTH DATE MM DD YY SEX M F
4. INSURED'S NAME (Last Name, First Name, Middle Initial)
5. PATIENT'S ADDRESS (No., Street)
6. PATIENT RELATIONSHIP TO INSURED Self Spouse Child Other
7. INSURED'S ADDRESS (No., Street)
CITY STATE
8. PATIENT STATUS Single Married Other
CITY STATE
ZIP CODE TELEPHONE (Include Area Code) ( )
Employed Full-Time Student Part-Time Student
ZIP CODE TELEPHONE (Include Area Code) ( )
9. OTHER INSURED'S NAME (Last Name, First Name, Middle Initial)
10. IS PATIENT'S CONDITION RELATED TO:
11. INSURED'S POLICY GROUP OR FECA NUMBER
a. OTHER INSURED'S POLICY OR GROUP NUMBER
a. EMPLOYMENT? (Current or Previous) YES NO
a. INSURED'S DATE OF BIRTH MM DD YY SEX M F
b. OTHER INSURED'S DATE OF BIRTH MM DD YY SEX M F
b. AUTO ACCIDENT? PLACE (State) YES NO
b. EMPLOYER'S NAME OR SCHOOL NAME
c. EMPLOYER'S NAME OR SCHOOL NAME
c. OTHER ACCIDENT? YES NO
c. INSURANCE PLAN NAME OR PROGRAM NAME
d. INSURANCE PLAN NAME OR PROGRAM NAME
10d. RESERVED FOR LOCAL USE
d. IS THERE ANOTHER HEALTH BENEFIT PLAN? YES NO If yes, return to and complete item 9 a-d.
READ BACK OF FORM BEFORE COMPLETING & SIGNING THIS FORM.
12. PATIENT'S OR AUTHORIZED PERSON'S SIGNATURE I authorize the release of any medical or other information necessary to process this claim. I also request payment of government benefits either to myself or to the party who accepts assignment below.
SIGNED DATE
13. INSURED'S OR AUTHORIZED PERSON'S SIGNATURE I authorize payment of medical benefits to the undersigned physician or supplier for services described below.
SIGNED
14. DATE OF CURRENT: MM DD YY ILLNESS (First symptom) OR INJURY (Accident) OR PREGNANCY(LMP)
15. IF PATIENT HAS HAD SAME OR SIMILAR ILLNESS. GIVE FIRST DATE MM DD YY
16. DATES PATIENT UNABLE TO WORK IN CURRENT OCCUPATION FROM TO
17. NAME OF REFERRING PROVIDER OR OTHER SOURCE
17a.
17b. NPI
18. HOSPITALIZATION DATES RELATED TO CURRENT SERVICES FROM TO
19. RESERVED FOR LOCAL USE
20. OUTSIDE LAB? YES NO $ CHARGES
21. DIAGNOSIS OR NATURE OF ILLNESS OR INJURY (Relate Items 1, 2, 3 or 4 to Item 24E by Line)
1. 2. 3. 4.
22. MEDICAID RESUBMISSION CODE ORIGINAL REF. NO.
23. PRIOR AUTHORIZATION NUMBER
24. A. DATE(S) OF SERVICE From To MM DD YY MM DD YY
B. PLACE OF SERVICE
C. EMG
D. PROCEDURES, SERVICES, OR SUPPLIES (Explain Unusual Circumstances) CPT/HCPCS MODIFIER
E. DIAGNOSIS POINTER
F. $ CHARGES
G. DAYS OR UNITS
H. EPSDT Family Plan
I. ID. QUAL.
J. RENDERING PROVIDER ID. #
1 NPI
2 NPI
3 NPI
4 NPI
5 NPI
6 NPI
25. FEDERAL TAX I.D. NUMBER SSN EIN
26. PATIENT'S ACCOUNT NO.
27. ACCEPT ASSIGNMENT? (For govt. claims, see back) YES NO
28. TOTAL CHARGE $
29. AMOUNT PAID $
30. BALANCE DUE $
31. SIGNATURE OF PHYSICIAN OR SUPPLIER INCLUDING DEGREES OR CREDENTIALS (I certify that the statements on the reverse apply to this bill and are made a part thereof.)
SIGNED DATE
32. SERVICE FACILITY LOCATION INFORMATION
a. NPI b.
33. BILLING PROVIDER INFO & PH # ( )
a. NPI b.
NUCC Instruction Manual available at: www.nucc.org
PLEASE PRINT OR TYPE
APPROVED OMB-0938-0999 FORM CMS-1500 (08-05)


**Figure 2-1:** The HCFA/CMS-1500 form.

## Determining whether medical billing is the right choice for you

Medical billers are responsible for billing insurance companies and patients correctly. As a biller, you need to understand how to read claim forms and payer explanation of benefits (EOBs); you need to understanding coding, even though you may not do that part of the job yourself; and you need to stay informed on the different claim submission standards for each payer you work with.

In addition, this job often requires daily interaction with both patients and insurance companies. The responsibility for explaining charges to patients may fall to the biller, particularly when patients need help understanding their payment obligations (such as co-insurance and copayments) per their policy. For that reason, billers need to have strong people skills both in person and on the telephone.

As a potential biller, keep in mind that working with patients can present a challenge. Often, they're sick or hurt during your interaction with them. Not only may they be contagious, but emotions may be high or minds may be fuzzy as well. Do your best to stay friendly and patient — and wash your hands frequently!

# In Tandem: Working Together or Doing Both Jobs Yourself?

Although you often hear people refer to billing and coding in the same breath — (see? I just did it ) — they're really two different jobs, as the preceding sections illustrate. After the coder has assigned the correct codes, the biller transforms the codes into a payable claim. As you pursue a career as a biller and coder, one of the things you should think about is whether you want to do both jobs or concentrate on just one. This decision may impact where you build your career, as I explain in the next sections.

## Wearing both hats

Both billing and coding job functions typically occur in the same office, whether on- or off-site. The flowchart in Figure 2-2 encapsulates the key functions that make up a combined billing and coding job.

Some physician practices keep their coding and billing in house, meaning it's done by their office staff. In these situations, there's no middle man, such as a practice management or billing company (discussed in the next section).

In some small practices, one person — the office coder/biller — does both jobs. This individual is the key to the business's accounts receivable. Anyone considering accepting this type of position should have experience in both areas and should possess a working knowledge of payer contracts, which you can read more about in Chapter 11.

If you want to do double duty as a coder/biller, be prepared for twice the work and being twice as vital to the success of your facility. Wearing both the billing hat and the coding hat makes you the one multitalented sheriff in town!

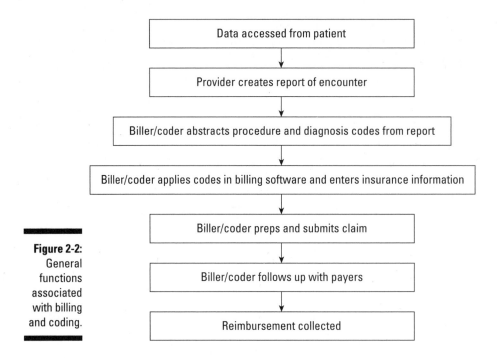

**Figure 2-2:**
General functions associated with billing and coding.

## Dedicating yourself to one job

The trend now is for physicians to use practice management or billing companies to facilitate their accounts receivables, and that makes billing companies a good place for a medical coder and biller to find work. These companies often employ several coders and billers, and it's definitely an environment in which you would do one job exclusively, due to the sheer volume of clients you service.

Billing companies often use various types of coding and billing software, and they offer the best opportunity to get experience in different systems, in addition to allowing the novice coder to learn from the more seasoned coders.

# Chapter 3

# Weighing Your Employment Options

*T*ranslating the work performed by the doctor and his staff into payment is known as the *revenue cycle*. The entire cycle involves coding the procedures according to the documentation, billing the procedures with the appropriate modifiers, sending the claim to the appropriate payer, and receiving payment from the insurance company and/or the patient.

The processes of billing and coding in that revenue cycle provide all sorts of job opportunities, from those in physician offices to hospitals to insurance companies and government payers. So the job of billing and coding is a far-reaching one that affords you myriad opportunities, which is good news as you determine what sort of professional setting you most prefer.

Regardless of where you end up, medical billing and coding is a profession that isn't going away anytime soon. In fact, thanks to recent government efforts to convert to electronic health records, the opportunities are growing. Where you choose to plant yourself is entirely up to you. So hop on the cycle! It's going to be a great ride.

# Choosing Your Environment: Doctor's Office, Hospital, and Others

Before you crack open the classifieds, give some thought to what sort of environment you want to work in. The possibilities are almost endless, and if you think about your preferences before you search for a job, you can narrow down your list of possible employers, saving yourself a boatload of time. Are you, for example, interested in the fast-paced, volume-heavy work that you'd likely find in a hospital? Or does the controlled chaos of a smaller physician's office seem more up your alley?

The good news is that all medical facilities and offices need some sort of billing and coding staff who can either work in the office or work remotely. Medical billers and coders are essential to the efficient processing of data, compliance with government regulations, and protection of patient privacy as required by the Health Insurance Portability and Accountability Act (HIPAA).

Currently, medical billing and coding jobs comprise one-fifth of the healthcare workforce, a number that is expected to grow. The transition to ICD-10, the updated version of the International Classification of Diseases that will replace ICD-9, is expected to increase the demand for medical coders because it will make the coding and billing process more complicated (due to the increased specificity of the classifications) and more time-consuming. ICD-10 is scheduled to go into effect in October 2014, and preparations for its roll-out are currently underway. You can read more about it in Chapter 15.

In the following sections, I outline several places that hire billers and coders.

As you consider where you want to ply your trade, keep in mind that the environment you choose can impact how broad or narrow your exposure to the coding and billing profession is. For example, if you work for a general surgeon (an optimal — and most sought after — position for a coder), you get experience in most areas of coding. The surgeon may use evaluation and management codes in addition to procedural codes from every section of the coding book. In contrast, a position in a pathology laboratory may limit your experience to that area of practice. A coder with experience in all areas becomes more valuable as an employee to the bigger employers.

## The doctor is in: Working in a physician's office

If you've seen someone buried under stacks of medical files as you take care of your copay in the doctor's office, chances are you're looking at a medical biller or coder. Just think — that could be you!

Several different kinds of physician offices employ their own coders and billers. Here are just a few possibilities:

- ✓ **Working in an office in which a group of physicians share a practice:** In a multi-physician office, the pace is usually a little faster, and more demands are placed on the administrative staff. Usually, a larger practice has an office manager in addition to the clerical staff.

- ✓ **Working in an office that has just one or two docs**: In this situation, the coder may function as the receptionist and biller as well. These offices can be great places to work. Due to size, you may find less office politics, and life usually tends to move at a slower pace when you're dealing with just one doc. The downside is that getting time off can be difficult, and your days off generally correspond to the physician's days off, so you have less flexibility with regard to personal time.

- ✓ **Working in an office in which the physicians do their own coding:** In this case, the physicians may use only the services of a biller. A certified coder is optimal to fill this type of position because, when the physician is out of his comfort zone from a coding perspective, a certified coder can assist with assigning the correct codes, as well as keeping abreast of code changes and other requirements. The downside to working in this environment is that your coding may not be as accurate as it should be (you may work with a physician who likes to "do it his way"), and moving to another job will be more difficult.

## Hooking up with a hospital

Get all the images of *Grey's Anatomy* of your head right now. Working in a hospital may be busy and exciting, but it's not always *that* dramatic, especially in the "back of house," where billers and coders do their stuff. That said, working in a hospital environment has a lot to keep you hopping.

Working in a hospital can be a rewarding experience for the coder. Hospitals are very departmentalized, with each department having its own coders. In most circumstances, the coding in a particular department is specific to a certain specialty or set of specialties, just as it would be if you were working in a physician's office. The difference is that the coding is for the facility, so expenses that are incurred by the facility — including drugs and implantable items (such as stints or shunts, for example) — are reimbursed through the hospital coding. In addition, most hospitals have a centralized billing department (or they may send the billing out to a billing company; see the next section).

Hospitals are reimbursed based on diagnosis-related groups (DRGs). This means that the admitting diagnosis is linked to the severity of the patient's illness. The level of risk associated with the treatment can affect the level of reimbursement received from Medicare and other payers. In other words, the sicker the patient, the greater the risk, and the higher the level of reimbursement.

Don't think that you can't create a niche for yourself in a larger hospital setting. You can, thanks to all the smaller sub-clinics and offices under the hospital umbrella that service the entire facility. For example, surgeries can't happen without anesthesia (well, they could, but it wouldn't be a popular choice!). So hospitals use anesthesiologists, who have to bill patients just like any other function of the hospital.

## Working at a billing or practice management company

Other options for employment as a biller or coder usually involve working for a practice management or billing company. These companies provide various levels of administrative support, with some handling all of a provider's practice administrative duties (even though having someone on site who understands insurance is still important for every provider office).

Billing and practice management companies come in all sizes and specialties. The larger companies handle numerous clients and usually have a team of people working on one or two of the accounts. In addition, if the company provides practice management — including coding and billing for a physician or group — the work is the same as if the provider were handling this aspect of the practice in-house.

Work at a billing or practice management company may be a good bet for the novice coder or biller because it's a great way to learn the ropes under the tutelage of a more seasoned professional. It also provides an outlet for giving and receiving feedback and working through some of the stickier details with a co-worker. In this work environment, you wouldn't be flying solo! As a general rule, bigger companies usually have more structure with regard to how they do things, and they provide the best on-the-job training.

Just as with hospitals, you can find your own niche in practice management companies, too. Some practice management companies within larger organizations, for example, specialize in certain areas, such as anesthesia or radiological practices. Working for one of these companies enables you to focus on and gain expertise in those specialties. With anesthesia, for example, you would need to know *all* surgical and procedural codes, and radiology overlaps with cardiology because of the non-invasive cardiac procedures that are now common.

Many billing companies are contractually obligated to their clients to employ only certified medical coders to perform the coding. Billers may often be trained on the job, but having knowledge prior to employment gives you an advantage as a job seeker.

## Working in claims for an insurance company

You may decide that you want to work in claims. Working in a claims job is one way to stretch the limits of your billing and coding knowledge.

Many insurance companies process their claims by computer. They either receive the information electronically or scan it into their processing software, where it is processed, ideally correctly. To ensure more efficient, yet timely, claim processing, many of these companies also use a claims processor.

To be successful as a claims processor, you need to know medical claim coding, billing procedures, and insurance obligations. These processors carefully examine each claim to determine its validity and accuracy. The processor then refers to the patient's insurance policy or plan to determine the level of processing for the claim. The processor also has software that contains the contracts that are linked to individual medical providers by their tax identification number or National Provider Identifier (NPI). They apply the claim to the plan provisions and payer contract to determine payment. After doing all this, the payment is issued accordingly. If the claim needs additional clarification or information, the claims processor sends a notice to the appropriate office to request the missing details.

In addition to payer-processing positions, insurance companies also need people to handle incorrectly processed claims when the providers appeal them. Again, solid knowledge of medical terminology, diagnosis, and procedural codes are valuable tools for these employees.

## The best of the rest

The possibilities are nearly endless in the billing and coding field. Even though you're most likely to find employment in a physician's office or in a larger facility like a hospital or clinic, here are just a few others you may find enticing:

- Nursing homes
- Outpatient facilities
- Home healthcare services
- Durable medical good providers
- Federal government agencies such as Health & Human Services, Social Security, Medicare, Tricare, or the Department of Labor

In short, billing and coding is important to any business that provides healthcare.

## Getting your foot in the door

Whether you find work in a doctor's office, at the local hospital, at a practice management company, or for an insurance company, you have several options for jobs within those offices. Think of the world of billing and coding as a buffet, and you have a plate just waiting to be filled with a big, tasty job. The good news is that you get to pick based on your level of skill and your interests.

 Still, finding employment as a novice can be a challenge. Many offices are fully staffed and may hesitate to hire a newly trained coder without any medical office experience. An excellent way to get your foot in the door is to accept a position that involves verifying each patient's benefits.

# Remote Access: Working Off-site

Working remotely — it's a good gig if you can get it! Some offices allow coders to work remotely. If you work off-site as a coder, you access the systems that contain the necessary documentation and then determine (or *abstract*) the correct diagnosis and procedural codes. You then return the codes to the billing department for claim submission.

In the following sections, I explain some of the things that make working remotely so enjoyable. But before you decide that working from home is for you, keep these important points in mind:

- ✔ **You must be able to ensure patient privacy.** When you work remotely, your office has less control over what you do and the environment in which you do it. For that reason, remote access places certain demands on you and the company to maintain HIPAA compliance. You must strictly follow policies and procedures to protect the privacy of the patients. For example, you need a private workspace that ensures that no one else — like guests and family members — can access patient information.

- ✔ **You must be able to work independently without supervision and still meet the company quotas that are normally imposed.** Companies that allow coders to work from home have the same expectations for their remote employees as they do for those working in the office. The remote worker normally is more productive if he or she exercises the same discipline that would be expected in the traditional office environment.

So take stock of your remote environment and your comfort level with shouldering that responsibility. If you feel comfortable that you can do both of the preceding, you may just find that working at home works for you!

## Working in your PJs

One obvious perk to working from home is the casual dress option. Many offices have relaxed dress codes, but only within the confines of your own home is working in a robe and slippers even an option.

As pleasant as that sounds, keep in mind that you may have to dress like a grown-up every now and again. Most companies still require remote coders to attend office meetings, workshops, and other professional functions. Plus, because you want your boss to be able to put a face to your name and because you want to make yourself available for questions from the billing department or follow-up people (divisions that are dependent upon the coder when questions arise in claim submission and processing), you'll probably head into the office on your own occasionally.

## The no-commute commute: Arranging a suitable workspace

One obvious perk to remote coding is that it eliminates the daily commute to an office, which saves energy, time, and money. The money you save on gas, clothes, lunches out, and wear and tear on your car (or a subway card) can go straight into the bank!

As a biller/coder, you need to make sure your workspace is equipped with a comfortable chair and a desk or table with room to spread out, a computer with Internet access, the appropriate software, and a telephone. Depending upon the company, you may also need a printer. In addition, you need the appropriate coding books.

Although some companies supply all the materials you need, including the paper and toner (and paying part of your Internet and phone bills), others expect you to provide these things on your own. Be sure to clarify the company's expectations as well as your own before entering into an agreement.

Some payers also allow people working in patient and provider support positions to work from home. Candidates for these positions must be able to maintain a professional demeanor from home, which means no barking dogs, crying babies, or other unprofessional background noises. If you have small children at home or you cannot secure a quiet room within your house (like a home office), then seriously consider setting up shop elsewhere. If, however, you've got a relatively quiet house during the day, then go for it!

# Looking at the downside of working remotely

Every silver lining has a cloud, and working remotely is no exception. Although it may be a wonderful solution for some, it's not a wonderful solution for all. In the next sections, I address some of the pitfalls.

### You don't get the benefits of being in the office

One downside to remote positions is that you have less interaction with co-workers. You may be the last to know when policies or procedures have changed. Working from home also does not offer the opportunity to cross-train in larger offices, which can affect your future employment options.

The employee with the most knowledge of office procedures and who is able to assist in other departments is a greater asset to the company. When you work remotely, you have fewer opportunities to prove your mettle within the office community. If you do choose to work remotely, try to find ways that you can keep that personal connection; otherwise, you may find yourself the first to be let go.

### The big "but": Generally not a good idea for the novice

Remote coding is for the seasoned professional, not for the novice — no matter what they tell you in TV commercials for technical schools. Initially you may think that abstracting billable procedural and diagnosis codes is clear-cut. It's not. Because many providers document in conversational format, coders often need clarification on what exactly was done. Experienced coders need less clarification and normally have developed a method for performing a physician query with finesse, thus allowing them to get the information they need.

When you work in an office, you have access to an experienced coder who can often assist you in understanding the verbiage in the documentation. If you're a newbie, consider putting off your remote access plans for a year or two until you have some office experience under your belt.

Part of your responsibility as a coder is to make sure that the documentation supports the claim being submitted for payment. If you're new to billing and coding, working in an office with the support of more experienced professionals can help you maintain that all-important accuracy. Think of it as a professional safety net. So if you do choose to fly the coop and ride solo, make sure you have strong support at the home office in case accuracy issues pop up.

# *Other Work Options: Freelance, Temping, and More*

A well-seasoned coder may carve out a reputation that enables him to work on his own in a freelance or consultant capacity. As a freelancer, you may be hired by companies for particular projects or by individual providers who need temporary help. As a consultant, you may assist the provider with hiring support staff and training the new staff in areas of claim billing and submission. In either case — when the project is finished or after the office is up and running — your work is done.

As a freelance or consultant coder, you find your own employment and contract for the specified duties to be performed. Freelancing is an option only for the expert coder who is fully capable of working independently.

Temporary work is another avenue sometimes taken by the experienced professional. Administrative staffing companies employ individuals for short- and long-term assignments. You register with the agency and go to the assignments offered to you. Sometimes offices need help replacing an employee on medical or disability leave. Although choosing this option may allow you to gain perspective on what type of work best suits you, often the employers are quite specific about the type of temporary help they need and usually require someone with some experience.

If you're new to billing and coding, freelancing, consultant coding, and temping are not good options for you, for the same reasons I outline in the earlier section "The big 'but': Generally not a good idea for the novice." If you need more convincing, read on.

# *A Word of Advice for New Coders*

As I mention earlier, working independently — whether you're working off-site, as a freelancer, as a consultant, or as a temp — isn't a good idea for a novice coder. The liability for errors is too much of a risk to both you and the provider.

Incorrect coding leads to incorrect billing, a situation sometimes known as *false claims reporting.* Fraudulent or false claims submission is a criminal act with serious penalties ranging from payment being taken back by a payer to imprisonment (if evidence of intent by the provider exists) to exclusion from federal programs.

Part of your job as a coder is to make sure that submitted claims are supported by the physicians' documentation. If the documentation does not support the claim and the error is discovered, the provider is liable for the incorrect payment and possibly additional repercussions. If the provider for whom you work is penalized, the next head to roll will likely be yours. Making this kind of error doesn't make for a good reference, and it presents a definite challenge in any future job interviews. So be proactive about ensuring that your coding is accurate! If you choose to freelance, remain in close contact with the physician's office and remember that no question is too small. Getting the answers you need from the doc can you save you, and her, a lot of hassle when bills are due.

The best thing you, as a novice coder, can do for yourself and future employers is to find work in a medical office, hospital, or billing company to gain experience in the medical profession. These environments introduce you to all areas of the claims process and make you more valuable to the company. In these environments, you learn the basics in a solid training program, and you learn the rest on the job. Physicians, if you work directly with them, and experienced coders can be wonderful mentors.

After you gain experience, you can branch out into alternative work scenarios. True, working in your PJs and having a 20-second commute from bedroom to home office is a lovely idea. But realize that you may have to pay some professional dues before your freelancing dreams can become a reality.

There is no substitute for experience. Exposure to the claims process and experienced billers and coders are the key to shaping you into a fully seasoned and very valuable coder yourself.

---

## Interning? Yes, please

Some vocational training schools work with local offices that allow students to do an internship. As an intern, you work in an office and are under direct supervision. Many offices have experienced coders and billers to serve as mentors. Sometimes, these opportunities evolve into regular employment. At a minimum, opportunities such as these give you experience and a professional reference.

Check with your school or professional organization about how to locate billing and coding internships in your area. Or check out the AAPC's Project Xtern program at www.aapc. com/medical-coding-jobs/project-xtern/index.aspx to find leads on internship opportunities.

# Part II

# Boning Up on the Need-to-Knows of Your Profession

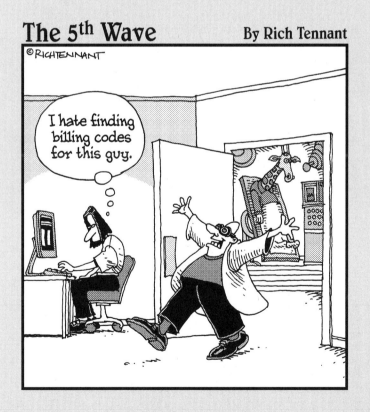

The 5th Wave          By Rich Tennant

©RICHTENNANT

I hate finding billing codes for this guy.

# In this part . . .

**D**ust off your security clearance because, as of now, you're on a need-to-know basis. And trust me, you really *do* need to know this stuff. This part is all about what you need to know to succeed in the medical billing and coding profession. I start by showing you the ins and outs of compliance, including what the rules are, who makes them, and how to make sure you follow them.

Other stuff on your need-to-know list includes a knowledge of medical terminology, an understanding of the concept of medical necessity, and a familiarity with the *payers* — the organizations that you'll deal with as you secure reimbursement for the provider.

# Chapter 4

# Compliance: Understanding the Rules

*C*ompliance — it's such a serious word, and for good reason. When people in the healthcare industry speak about compliance by healthcare providers, they mean that an office or individual has set up a program to run the practice according to the regulations set forth by the United States Office of Inspector General (OIG). Yep, pretty serious, indeed. The regulations are designed to prevent fraud and abuse by healthcare providers, and as a medical biller or coder, you must familiarize yourself with the basics of compliance.

Not only must you follow rules regarding how to process and bill claims, but you must also follow rules regarding the confidentiality of healthcare information. You can thank something called the Health Insurance Portability and Accountability Act (HIPAA) for setting the bar for compliance. This act was passed by Congress in 1996 and is sometimes called the Privacy Rule. It established the first national standard for use and disclosure of health information and guarantees certain rights to individuals with regard to their healthcare. HIPAA outlines how certain entities (health plan, clearinghouse, or healthcare provider, for example) can use or disclose personal health information, or PHI. In addition, under HIPAA, patients must be allowed access to their medical records.

In this chapter, I tell you who the key rule makers are and explain how you can stay on the right side of the law.

# You Rule! Getting to Know the Rule Makers

The rule-making game has several players, and most of them are somehow related to good old Uncle Sam. The United States Department of Health & Human Services (HHS) is the primary U.S. government agency responsible for protecting the health of Americans. Medicare and Medicaid, part of the Centers for Medicare & Medicaid Services (CMS), are two of this agency's programs, and together they provide healthcare insurance for millions of Americans. This department's programs serve the U.S.'s most vulnerable citizens.

The OIG protects the operations of the HHS. This oversight also extends to programs under other HHS institutions, including the Centers for Disease Control and Prevention (CDC), National Institutes of Health (NIH), and the Food and Drug Administration (FDA).

The American Medical Association (AMA), which develops, maintains, and owns the copyright to CPT codes, determines what the code represents. The CMS works with the AMA to determine correct coding edits and which codes are incidental to others.

As a biller and coder, you need to be familiar with these organizations. The following sections outline the key organizations that you'll work with as a medical biller and coder.

## The Centers for Medicare & Medicaid Services (CMS)

As mentioned previously, the Centers for Medicare & Medicaid Services (CMS) is the home of two government healthcare programs: Medicare and Medicaid.

Originally, Medicare was intended to provide healthcare to the elderly at the age of 65. In the years that followed, the need for access to healthcare for others, including children, the disabled, and those with certain illnesses, became apparent. Today, Medicare also includes those with physical or mental disabilities and those awaiting organ transplants, as well as prescription drug coverage.

Because these programs serve so many Americans and use taxpayer dollars to do so, the government has established rules governing what services are covered, the acceptable level of compensation for the service providers, and how claims should be processed.

Medicare policies regarding medical necessity, frequency of procedures, and other payment rules are often used as guidelines for commercial payers as well. For complete information about the policies for Medicare claims processing, check out the Internet-only manuals on the CMS website (www.cms.gov).

Medicare policy rules change pretty frequently, and they affect payment for certain procedures. Take a procedure as simple as a lesion excision (removing a cyst or skin growth), for example. Medicare pays for this procedure only under a specific set of rules (the diagnoses must support medical necessity). If the rules regarding this procedure change, and if these changes affect your employer, it may be your job as a coder job to keep the physician or staff informed.

## The Office of Inspector General (OIG)

The Office of Inspector General (OIG) was established in 1976 to oversee programs administered through HHS. Much of the OIG's efforts focus on identifying waste, fraud, and abuse in Medicare, Medicaid, and other federal programs.

The branch of the OIG associated with HHS is the largest inspector general office in the federal government. These efforts are necessary because of the significant amount of money needed to finance these programs and the sheer number of citizens they serve.

The OIG conducts audits and tracks how government funds are spent. The findings of these investigations are often the foundation for Medicare or Medicaid policy changes and procedural code changes initiated by CMS or the AMA. The OIG publishes the results of its investigation on its website (http://oig.hhs.gov).

Even though most of these government organizations are sole entities, they typically rely on each other in one way or another. For example, because developments in medical technology and treatment options are usually far ahead of legislation, Medicare often discovers through an OIG investigation that taxpayer funds are not being used efficiently.

## The individual payer (insurance company)

When you hear the term *individual payers,* you may assume it refers to individuals, but it doesn't. Individual payers are actually the insurance companies that provide group and individual coverage plans to your patients. Each payer has its own policies and procedures, which are published and available for both patients and providers to review. The payer may be a plan administrator that is part of a pricing network or may serve as administrator for sponsored plans.

More often than not, CMS sets the bar when it comes to payer rules. As I mention earlier, Medicare follows a strict set of claims-processing policies that include correct coding edits, mutually exclusive procedures edits, modifier requirements, unit requirements, and numerous other specifications. In addition, Medicare allows claims to be submitted within 12 months. Individual payers may follow the Medicare rules for payment, but they don't *have* to follow them. In fact, many often have their own policies.

Individual payers employ their own processing policies, including which edits they follow, which modifiers they recognize, and other payer-specific rules. As the coder and biller, you must be knowledgeable about each payer's policies when you prepare a claim for submission. If you don't follow the payer's policies, the claim may pay incorrectly or not at all.

In addition, most commercial payers have much shorter timely filing requirements than Medicare's 1-year limit, usually 90 days — which isn't a long time when crucial documentation is missing!

# Complying with HIPAA

Strict regulations are necessary in billing and processing medical claims because the opportunity for fraud and abuse is ever present on both sides. The Health Insurance Portability and Accountability Act (HIPAA), passed by Congress in 1996, set a national standard for protecting health data and protecting the patient's rights.

Before HIPAA, individual state laws governed the privacy of health information, and these laws often varied from state to state. Under HIPAA, providers, plans, and all healthcare services must comply with federal standards. In addition, individual states still have the authority to set guidelines; they may be more stringent than the national standard, but they cannot be more lenient.

Here are the key provisions of HIPAA:

✔ **HIPAA guarantees everyone a basic right to privacy in addition to the right to have access to his or her own medical records.** Providers may charge a reasonable fee for access to the records and also may adopt policies with regard to compliance (for example, the process patients must follow to request records, or how the office is structured to ensure patient confidentiality).

✔ **HIPAA requires that all providers must inform their patients of their privacy practices.** These notices include a disclosure about how medical information is used and the patient's right to file a complaint with the Department of Health & Human Services Office of Civil Rights.

As a general rule, personal health information (PHI) can be disclosed only with the consent of the patient. However, in some instances, PHI may be shared without the consent of the patient. Such circumstances include those that benefit the public, such as certain communicable diseases that must be reported to the CDC, records that are under subpoena in criminal cases, and the like.

✔ **HIPAA gives patients the right to know who has accessed their health records within the prior six years.** This disclaimer, however, doesn't need to include the people and other entities (such as clearinghouses and billing services) who see the records during the daily task of patient care. In other words, you don't need to let the patient know which clearinghouse the office uses, whether billing is outsourced, or other such practice information.

Organizations that are not bound by HIPAA rules include life insurance companies, Workers' Compensation companies, Social Security agencies, law enforcement agencies, researchers who are provided information by healthcare providers, companies that offer screenings at malls, and other such entities. Entities who are covered by HIPAA are responsible for implementing a compliance plan.

Under HIPAA, all reported breaches of compliance regulations must be investigated, and violators may face civil or criminal penalties. For that reason, it is essential that all cogs of the healthcare industry (including you as a biller and coder) be familiar with HIPAA rules.

---

# The 411 on the EHR

EHR stands for *electronic health record*. The future of medicine is the EHR. Use of the electronic records is intended to do away with the paper chart and make protecting and sharing information easier for providers. If a physician has access to the hospital's records, he or she can receive test results, pathology reports, and other information needed to treat the patient immediately.

EHRs are also considered to be more secure. They're password protected and can be programmed so that even those who have access to the records don't have access to the entire record, but only those parts necessary to do their jobs. The front office, for example, may need full access to patient demographics and insurance information, but it may not need access to test results. Similarly, the nurse caring for the patient needs full access to health information but probably doesn't need to know the patient's Social Security number or address.

## Going beyond HIPAA's confidentiality rules

HIPAA does more than simply deal with confidentiality:

✔ Title I of HIPAA protects health insurance coverage for workers and their families who change or lose their jobs. Under HIPAA, a new group health insurance must accept most of the medical conditions that were covered by a patient's previous group policy. When an individual enrolls in a new group health plan, the plan may refuse to cover certain defined conditions for a period of 12 to 18 months. This exclusion is reduced by the amount of time that the patient had coverage under his or her previous group health plan. As the biller or coder, you must know this rule so that you can challenge an unlawful pre-existing denial by a commercial payer.

✔ Title II of HIPAA requires a national standard for electronic transactions and national identifiers for providers, insurers, and employers. These identifiers are known as Tax ID (similar to an individual's Social Security number) and National Provider Identification (NPI) numbers. Payers have payer identification numbers called payer IDs, 5-digit numbers that identify to which payer a claim is to be sent electronically. As a medical biller or coder, you must know and follow these standards to avoid violations for which your employer will be held accountable. (This is also the clause that contains the standards used to ensure the privacy of health information.)

✔ Title III of HIPAA addresses the way employers handle medical savings accounts, which are tax-deferred savings accounts that are used only to cover medical expenses.

✔ Title IV of HIPAA mandates that employers must allow employees to continue their health insurance when taking a new job.

✔ Title V of HIPAA provides employers with ways to offset the cost of compliance, such as deducting life-insurance premiums from their tax returns.

## *Doing your part: Do's and don'ts of compliance*

Even though HIPAA has changed privacy and data protection for the better, don't be fooled into thinking that information that should be held confidential between doctor and patient stays in the examination room. Patient information is exchanged in many places, so discretion on the part of all staff is imperative to protect the rights of your patients.

Consider this: In earlier days, patient charts were kept in file cabinets or record rooms. Ideally, only those with a need to see those records were allowed access. Today, because of electronic data transfer, all patient information finds its way into data files. Without high levels of security, confidential patient information could easily find its way into the wrong hands.

Ultimately, all employees (this means you, too) within an organization bound by HIPAA are responsible for maintaining compliance to the best of their abilities. With regard to patient confidentiality, the general idea is really simple: Those who do not need to know should not be told. Patients in the waiting room do not need to know anything about another patient. They don't need to know another patient's name, address, phone number, Social Security number, birth date, or any other personal information. Nor do they need to know why that patient is there. Your office should have a process that allows every patient to relay this information without anyone else in attendance being privy to that info.

Your employer is responsible for having a compliance implementation plan and a way to monitor whether the plan is being followed. In small offices, one individual may be responsible for monitoring practices, like making sure computers are password protected, making sure that sensitive areas are secure, and so on. Larger facilities normally have a number of people monitoring compliance within the practice. These individuals include informational technology specialists who make sure that no software viruses or network breaches occur.

You also have an important role to play. Fortunately, the do's and don'ts of compliance are basic.

Here are the things on your Do list:

- ✔ Treat patients' personal information as you would like your own information to be treated: Keep it secure and respect their right to privacy.

- ✔ Use passwords that are not obvious (*password* is not a password; neither is *12345*), keep them in a secure place that is also password protected, and change them regularly.

- ✔ If you need to be in patient areas, be discreet. If you work in a surgery center, wear the uniform so that patients are not uncomfortable with a stranger in street clothes.

- ✔ Keep your voice down when discussing patient finances, both in person and over the phone.

- ✔ Be professional at all times.

And here are the don'ts:

- ✔ Don't write your passwords on the side of your computer, share the passwords with other staff members for their use, or use the same password for everything. (Note that most office policies require that all passwords be registered with either the office manager or compliance officer; that's fine.)

- ✔ Don't discuss personal issues in the presence of patients.

In many offices, the coder is the one with the best resources for staying abreast of compliance regulations. These issues are often discussed at local chapter meetings, and they're the subject of articles in professional publications. The coder also needs to stay aware of Medicare policies, which include compliance issues.

Beyond your official responsibilities regarding compliance, keep in mind that, as part of the office staff, you can help guard confidentiality in other ways. For example, family members of the office staff don't belong in the secure areas of the office, and visitors to the office need to identify themselves and the reason for their visit. If you see people in areas they shouldn't be in, inquire why they're there and direct them elsewhere. (*Note:* Every office needs a form that obligates visitors to register and sign that they agree to protect any patient information that unintentionally finds its way to them.)

## Uh-oh! Consequences of non-compliance

Violating HIPAA is referred to as *non-compliance*. When HIPAA has been violated, the provider is subject to a fine and is responsible for fixing the problem.

Even accidentally or unintentionally releasing protected information is a HIPAA violation. This type of violation varies in the level of severity, and the minimum penalty is $100, but if the violation is repeated, the fine can increase to several thousands of dollars. If the unintentional violation was a result of neglect and the provider doesn't take steps to correct the problem, the fine can rise to more than $1 million.

The penalties for intentional violations are even worse. Intentionally releasing protected information results in higher fines and may include a jail sentence. If the information is released for financial gain or malice, jail time may be up to 10 years and include a stiff fine.

To read more about possible repercussions of privacy violations, go to the HHS website (www.hhs.gov/ocr/privacy/hipaa/understanding/summary/index.html).

## Unbundling the Compliance Bundle

Compliance rules also relate to billing practice. Being in compliance with billing practice means working within the correct coding edits (the NCCI edits). *NCCI* stands for National Correct Coding Initiative, which stipulates that, when you're coding multiple procedures, the extra procedure coded should have required that the physician perform extra work that is not normally part of the procedure.

The revenue cycle starts with the codes, and they must be the correct codes. Every CPT code represents a potential reimbursement, and you don't want payers making payment under false circumstances. But you do want the physician to be paid for the work he has done.

## Looking at incidental procedures

Certain procedures are considered *incidental* to another procedure; that is, one procedure could not be completed without the other procedure and is, therefore, not a separate billable procedure. The edits usually indicate that. When you check procedural codes, you see incidental procedures reflected as *bundled*, which means they're *inclusive* to another procedure. In other words, if a second or even third procedure is done through the same incision, the incidental procedure may not justify extra reimbursement.

That doesn't mean the provider can't get paid for additional work, however. When a procedure takes an extraordinarily long time or requires more than the accepted standard of work, you can apply a certain modifier, which may earn the physician additional reimbursement.

Other times, you can unbundle the procedure. When you unbundle, you include additional codes on the claim to represent procedures that, although incidental to the primary procedure, actually merit additional reimbursement. The next sections give you the details.

## When unbundling's okay

Sometimes, unbundling is supported. For example, if the provider performs a procedure that is listed as inclusive but does so through a separate incision, you can unbundle the codes. Perhaps the surgeon is working on more than one part of the body. If she performs a left knee meniscectomy (removing all or part of the *meniscus,* the pad of cartilage) and a right knee chondroplasty (shaving the cartilage), you'd unbundle the chondroplasty, even though a chondroplasty is always considered incidental to a meniscectomy. Why? Because it's obviously not incidental when it's performed on a different leg.

The edits are there for a reason: Unbundling procedures isn't always okay. In fact, it's often *not* okay. So how do you know what the edits are? You can find the Correct Coding Initiative (CCI) edits on the CMS website and in most coding software programs. These programs are a good investment for most companies that bill surgeries, partly because they let the coder know when unbundling procedures is okay. Keep in mind, though, that some payers use their own editing programs that differ from the CMS version. If your employer is contracted with a payer, the contract usually defines which set of edits to follow. Certain medical associations also have their own ideas about procedures that may or not be incidental to the main procedure.

In general, follow the CMS edits; if the payer says to do otherwise, then follow the contract.

## When bundling's not okay

Unbundling for the sole purpose of billing a higher dollar amount on a claim is never okay. Before procedures can be considered for additional payment, the physician must document the extra work. This documentation must be very specific and meet the guidelines for unbundling as outlined in the editing software and coding materials.

If something is unbundled incorrectly and the claim is audited by the payer, the physician or provider is obligated to return payment. In some instances, the payer may terminate the provider's contract. The payer may also ask for interest on wrongfully paid claims.

## Defining exclusivity

*Exclusivity* means that one procedure is not possible under specific circumstances. Some procedures are gender specific, and other procedures are not possible under certain circumstances. Read on for the details.

### Understanding mutually exclusive procedures

Mutually exclusive procedures fall into two categories:

- ✔ **A procedure that can't be done in combination with another:** Because some procedures can't be successfully performed together, they are not going to be paid on the same claim. Here's an example (albeit an extreme one that helps explain the concept): Imagine that the patient has suffered severe damage to his arm. During surgery, the surgeon tries but fails to repair the arm and decides that amputation is necessary. You can't code for both a fracture repair and an amputation if both occurred during the same session. Nor is the insurance company going to pay for both the fracture repair and amputation in this situation. If the amputation was deemed necessary, then that is the procedure you code and bill for.

    However, if the physician repaired the fracture and then three weeks later the patient returned with severe necrosis (tissue death) and was becoming septic — a life-endangering condition — then the provider can bill both procedures.

- ✔ **Procedures that are not possible under the present circumstances:** This type of exclusivity relates to procedures that are age- or sex-related. Men do not give birth. Women do not have prostate procedures. Exclusivity may be defined as not possible under the presented circumstances.

### *Understanding contractual exclusions*

Exclusivity may be a reference to procedures, as explained in the preceding section, or it may relate to contractual terms. Payer contracts may pertain to the type of plan — Health Maintenance Organization (HMO) or Preferred Provider Organization (PPO), for example — sponsored by that company. Each plan has different payment obligations that must be met for a claim to be paid.

HMOs, for example, require the patient to name a primary care physician (PCP) who acts as a gatekeeper for spending the insurance company's money. The patient is required to seek treatment from the PCP first. If that physician feels that the illness or injury requires the services of a specialist, then he may refer the patient to a specialist within the network.

Exclusivity may also refer to the network. Some plans do not allow patients to see out-of-network or non-contract providers. Their coverage is exclusive to providers within the network. PPOs, for example, normally allow the patient to visit any provider that is contracted with the insurance company. If the patient visits a non-contracted provider, the claim is considered *out-of-network*, and the plan may pay for the services but at a much higher cost to the patient.

Contracts between payers and providers may contain fee schedules or payment agreements that are exclusive to various plans within their organization. These agreements are exclusive to the terms of the contract. They apply only to a certain payer under defined conditions, and claims must be filed within the terms defined in the contract(s).

## Symbolizing coding

Coding books have symbols that serve as reminders with respect to the codes. They have symbols that indicate the number of digits in a diagnosis code. They have symbols that tell the coder whether the procedure is considered *unilateral* (one-sided). They indicate whether the procedure is covered per Medicare regulations. They have symbols for female, male, and numerous other specifications. Other symbols alert the coder whether a code was added, changed, or may have been deleted at the beginning of the current year (a good reason to make sure you are using a current edition of CPT and ICD.)

The coding books, together with Medicare and payer websites, guide you when you abstract information from the medical record. Keeping current on code changes, regulatory guidelines, and legislation will keep the revenue cycle in motion and maintain the provider's compliance with both billing regulations and privacy obligations.

# Fun with Audits — Not Really

In the event of an audit by the payer, an internal auditor, or an external auditor, an auditing coder (someone just like you) recodes the audited claims. In doing so, he or she should be able to abstract the same information from the record documentation that you did. If the audit comes back with a different code, an explanation for the difference accompanies the audit. That discrepancy could be the result of a couple of things:

- ✔ A recent change in coding rules that you were unaware of.
- ✔ You missed certain codes.

If so, use the audit as a learning experience. But if the auditor sees a different code entirely or misses a code that you submitted, challenge the audit and explain your reason for coding the claim the way you did. The auditor may agree to your position or may be able to explain the flaw in your reasoning.

Regardless of the differences, audits are about improving. They help you grow and improve as a coder, and they reiterate to the provider the importance of documenting procedures correctly. If the physicians you work for questions your skill as a coder because you didn't fare well in an audit, ask to be allowed to attend a practice-specific workshop or webinar to help you become a better employee.

## Understanding the difference between internal and payer audits

Several different kinds of billing and coding audits exist, but all refer to an independent review conducted by a different person with coding background to verify the accuracy of your work. Providers conduct audits because, although they don't like to leave money on the table, they don't want to be paid more than they deserve.

Most large companies have an internal auditing department, whose auditors randomly select charts to evaluate. Other providers, usually smaller ones, send quarterly audits to an outside consulting firm. The auditors look for under-coding, over-coding, and incorrect coding. Often, if an error is found during an audit, the result is to submit a corrected claim, possibly with a copy of the medical record and a letter explaining the reason for the request.

Other audits are *payer audits.* Most payer contracts contain a clause that allows the payer to request medical records, invoices, and other supporting documentation for claims paid within the past year (or, in some instances, farther back). Medicare is a payer that can just show up and request to see records on site. Payer audits are performed to verify that claims submitted for reimbursement have the necessary supporting documentation, such as invoices, procedure notes, or test results.

Currently a bit of publicity has surrounded the Medicare RAC audits, which are being conducted by Medicare's Recovery Audit Contractors. The RAC audits are a result of the 2003 Medicare Modernization Act. As a result of this legislation, CMS and RAC auditors recouped more than $980 million from providers in the three initial states of Florida, New York, and California. The objective of the RAC audit differs from a traditional Medicare audit in several ways. First, the RAC auditors are essentially functioning as bounty hunters and are paid a commission equal to 10 percent of the amount recouped. The audits focus on CMS payment criteria, such as medical necessity relative to procedures. The RAC auditors also examine compliance with Medicare's payment criteria, documentation, and billing requirements.

## Avoiding an audit: You can't

Audits are a necessary evil because they are usually the only system that enables a company to keep tab on its coders. Normally, when you pay for a service, you see the end result, but not the insurers. Instead, these payers entrust the providers with the power to simply send a form and declare that the work was done. Audits keep everyone on their toes, which can only be good for both sides. Also keep in mind that when payers, especially Medicare, recoup money, they often ask for interest.

Bottom line: Audits are unavoidable, but they don't have to be miserable. In the next section, I explain how to ensure that the auditors don't find problems with your work.

## Protecting yourself from an audit

If the documentation is clear, an audit is no problem, and documentation is the only way to protect yourself in an audit. Follow this advice:

- ✔ Make sure you understand the documentation needed to code and bill procedures.

- ✔ Make sure that you understand the payer contracts and submit claims within the confines of that contract.

- ✔ Be especially careful with unbundling. Codes are bundled for a reason: because they should be included with the primary procedure that was performed. Sometimes, procedures are extra, usually for anatomical reasons. Then, coding both procedures separately may be okay, but make certain that the documentation supports both procedures.

✔ Make sure that you code only what the documentation supports and that everything you do as a coder is part of the record. The phrase "That is what the doctor meant" can be a problem for obvious reasons. If a provider insists that, when he says "A," he means "B," then get it in writing. The same holds true for unbundling procedures. If the provider insists that certain procedures be submitted "because he wants to track them" or because "XYZ will pay it," *get it in writing.*

If you follow these guidelines, you can stop sweating and start getting your ducks in a row so you're prepared if and when the time comes to have your work audited. That way, you have no worries.

# Chapter 5

# Not-So-Strange Bedfellows: Medical Terminology and Medical Necessity

. . . . . . . . . . . . . . . . . . . . . . . . . . . . . . . . . . . . . . . . . . .

*In This Chapter*

▶ Working your way through basic anatomy

▶ Getting familiar with medical terminology

▶ Defining different procedure types

▶ Navigating the world of patient evaluation and management

. . . . . . . . . . . . . . . . . . . . . . . . . . . . . . . . . . . . . . . . . . .

*1*n billing and coding, you've got to know as much about the language that helps create all those billing codes as you do about how to perform the coding. Two big building blocks help construct the basis for billing and coding: medical terminology and medical necessity.

*Medical terminology* refers to the words that describe illness, injury, conditions, and procedures. The majority of the word parts that make up medical terms originate in Greek and Latin. *Medical necessity* refers to the requirement that any procedures performed are necessary to diagnose or treat a medical condition while maintaining an acceptable standard of care. A whole group of other terms, called *diagnosis terms,* are the basis for the codes you enter to substantiate medical necessity.

Insurance companies are usually the parties responsible for paying the healthcare provider for services rendered. However, an insurance company pays only for procedures that are medically necessary to the well-being of the patient, its client. For that reason you must link each procedure billed to a diagnosis that supports the medical necessity for the procedure. All diagnosis and procedures are worded in medical terminology. To accurately abstract (or identify) the correct codes, you must understand the verbiage used in the record, as well as surgical procedures and care and management procedures. This chapter tells you what you need to know.

# Basic Anatomy Does a Body Good

The first class in most coding programs is a human anatomy class. *Anatomy* is the study of the human body structure. Anatomy is broken down into sub-topics, including *gross anatomy,* which relates to the part of the body that can be seen.

Typical coding programs educate you in all areas of anatomy from the out-side in, with a particular focus on the disease process and its effect on how the body functions. *Disease process* is defined as a deviation of the normal structure or function of a body part that is represented by symptoms.

In the following sections, I give you a crash course in body systems, illness and disease, and injuries.

The disease process doesn't occur in a vacuum. It always affects a specific body system, which itself is made up of particular organs. As the coder, you need to understand the disease process as it relates to procedures to be billed. The diagnosis code (insurance speak for medical necessity) rep-resents the disease or injury. The diagnosis code that's linked to the proce-dure must show the necessity of the procedure being billed. You can find the procedure code in the appropriate section of the Current Procedural Terminology (CPT) book.

## Getting familiar with body systems

A *body system* is a group of organs that perform a specific task. For example, the nervous system includes the brain, the spinal cord, and the nerves.

Information about body systems matters to you because coding books are structured according to the body systems. The books that you'll use are known as CPT books, which, for the most part, contain all the procedural codes you can bill. These books contain the procedures as defined by the American Medical Association (AMA), and they're updated each year; some codes are added, and some are deleted. The new codes usually become effective on January 1. So make sure that you always use the most current edition!

Table 5-1 lists the major body systems you'll likely encounter on the job (and in your CPT books in the section devoted to that system).

| Table 5-1 | Major Body Systems |
|---|---|
| *System* | *Organs Involved* |
| Cardiovascular | Blood vessels, heart, and lymph system |
| Digestive | Structures inside the mouth, stomach, and colon, all the way down to the rectum |
| Endocrine | Thyroid, parathyroid, and adrenal glands |
| Eye and ocular adnexa and auditory | Eyes and ears |
| Female genital (see note) | Ovaries, fallopian tubes, uterus, and external genitalia |
| Integument | Skin and nails |
| Male genital (see note) | Penis, prostrate, testes |
| Musculoskeletal | Connective tissue, muscles, ligaments, and bones |
| Nervous | Brain, spinal cord, and nerves |
| Respiratory | Airway and lungs |
| Urinary (see note) | Kidneys, bladder, ureters, and urethra |

**Note:** *In some reference books, the male and female urinary systems are combined with the urinary system and referred to as the genito-urinary system.*

After you identify the correct system code from the CPT, your next step is to find the supporting diagnosis codes for the procedures. You can find these in the ICD-9 book (International Classification of Diseases, Ninth Edition). Lucky for you, the ICD-9 book also categorizes diagnosis codes by body system (in addition to other sections that contain codes for illness and other non-specific codes).

In October 2014, the United States will start reporting disease and injury using ICD-10 codes. You can read more about ICD-9 and ICD-10 in Chapter 15.

After you're familiar with the basic body systems, it's time to think about what can go wrong with them. When a system is not functioning properly, an illness or disease process is at work.

## Getting a handle on illness and disease

Most of the codes that you encounter as a biller/coder have something to do with a patient's illness. *Illness* is a catch-all term that refers to a feeling or condition of not being healthy. Although an illness may be due to a disease, a disease has measurable symptoms, and it affects normal body functions.

Be sure that you know the difference between *illness* and *disease*. Just as you may be ill but not be suffering from a disease, you may be suffering from a disease but not feel ill. A patient may have influenza, an illness, for example, but that doesn't mean she's suffering from a disease. Conversely, a patient may have Type 2 diabetes, a disease, but she may not feel bad or be experiencing obvious symptoms.

During a patient encounter, the physician examines the patient, documents his findings, and then determines the best course of action for treatment. When performing this type of service, the physician bills for an evaluation and management encounter (also known as an *E&M visit*), which is a fancy way of referring to a doctor's visit, or a *consultation* (a visit requested by another physician or healthcare entity). Whether a physician conducts an E&M visit or a consultation, he or she will report some sort of illness or disease-related term in the patient's record, even if the problem is something as simple as the common cold. (You can read more about E&M and consultation visits in the later sections "Connecting with the world of Evaluation and Management Codes" and "Dealing with Consultation Visits.")

## Dealing with injuries

Many physician encounters are due to injury, and the difference between disease and injury can be blurred. A patient may suffer bruising due to disease, for example, but have no history of injury. This is why, for the purposes of coding, you want to be familiar with the varying levels of injury:

- ✔ **Acute injury:** Damage to the body incurred by accident
- ✔ **Chronic injury:** Damage to the body that is a result of overuse or aging

Treatment may differ depending upon whether the injury is acute or chronic. With an acute injury, the injury has just happened, and the tissue in question is still viable. A chronic injury, on the other hand, has occurred over time or is a once-acute injury that has only partially healed. Often, treatment of a chronic injury requires additional work: A surgeon may need to remove nonviable tissue or possibly use tissue grafts to successfully complete the repair. Thus, a chronic injury is often more time-consuming because the body's tendency to heal itself can result in scar tissue (called *fibrosis*).

If you have any question about whether the injury is acute or chronic, investigate further before choosing a procedure code. If the patient history is available for review, you can abstract the information you need to choose the correct code. In this case, you would review the patient history to see when the patient first came in for treatment, or you would look for the patient information page to see whether the patient indicated when the injury occurred.

Many times, patients say that they have no idea why the problem occurred. In this situation, you probably have to use chronic injury-related codes unless the provider says otherwise.

Because the story may be more complicated than a one-time incident, don't assume that an injury is acute. When you're unsure, investigate. Check for clues in the report. For example, words such as *pathological* often indicate a disease process that would point to chronic, not acute, injury.

# Say What? Deciphering Medical Terminology

Anatomy, illness, injury, and disease are all based in specific medical language and terms. By deciphering the medical terminology used in medical records, you can more easily assign the correct diagnosis and procedural codes. For that reason, a solid foundation in medical terminology is essential for the coder.

A whole world of medical terminology is out there for you to explore, and solid coding programs offer classes in medical terminology. In this section, I take you on a quick tour of the terminology you need to know. (For more detailed information, take a look at *Medical Terminology For Dummies,* by Beverley Henderson and Jennifer Lee Dorsey [Wiley].)

 Most medical terms are two-parters; that is, they're made up of prefixes and suffixes. Some medical terms also have a word segment in the middle, but the majority of medical terms are built with the prefix/suffix combination. These word parts are almost always Greek or Latin in origin. If you have a background in these languages (or have studied words derived from Greek or Latin), you'll have a great head start in understanding medical terminology.

## In the beginning: Knowing your prefixes

A *prefix* refers to the beginning segment of the word. The prefix of the word often is the first clue about which body part or which area the procedure relates to. Some examples of prefixes are *arthr(o)-* (joint), *hemi-* (half), *cardi-* (heart), and *bronch-* (air, airway). When you see a word beginning with *arthro-* (for example, *arthroscopy*), you know that it has something to do with the joint. Similarly, *bronchoscopy* has something to do with the airway (in the next section, I explain what the suffixes, or word endings, mean). Table 5-2 lists some of the more common prefixes.

| Table 5-2 | Common Greek and Latin Prefixes | | |
|---|---|---|---|
| **Prefix** | **Meaning** | **Prefix** | **Meaning** |
| a- | Absent or lack of | hyper- | Above |
| ab- | Away from | hypo- | Under |
| abdomino- | Referring to the abdomen | hyster- | Pertaining to the uterus |
| alb- | White | inter- | Among |
| ad- | Away from | intra- | Inside |
| angi- | Pertaining to vessels | leuko- | White |
| ante- | Before | macro- | Large |
| anti- | Against | micro- | Small |
| arthr(o)- | Joint | my(o)- | Muscle |
| aud- | Hearing | necro- | Dead |
| auto- | Self | neo- | New |
| brady- | Slow | nephro- | Kidney |
| bronch- | Air, airway | neuro- | Nerve |
| calc- | Stone | osteo- | Bone |
| cardi- | Heart | path- | Disease |
| cerebro- | Brain | sarc- | Flesh |
| chondr- | Cartilage | sub- | Under |
| circum- | Around | super- | Above |
| derm- | Skin | teno- | Tendon |
| dys- | Painful, difficult | tachy- | Fast |
| entero- | Intestine | thrombo- | Clot |
| gastro- | Of the stomach | trans- | Across |
| hemi- | Half | trich- | Hair |
| hepat- | Liver | | |

## Sussing out the suffixes

The terms you encounter in the coding world have to end somehow, and that happens with a suffix, which has a special meaning all its own. *Suffixes* describe condition or action. For example, *-scopy* means to use an instrument to view. Therefore, you know that the word *arthroscopy* refers to looking into the joint with a scope (the prefix *arthro-* refers to the joint), and *bronchoscopy* refers to looking into the airway (*bronch-* means "air") with a scope. (Refer to the preceding section for common medical prefixes.)

Table 5-3 lists common suffixes and their meanings.

| Table 5-3 | Common Greek and Latin Suffixes | | |
|-----------|---------------------------------|-----------|---------|
| **Suffix** | **Meaning** | **Suffix** | **Meaning** |
| -algia | Pain | -ostomy | Opening |
| -asis | Condition or state of | -pathy | Disease |
| -cide | Destroy | -penia | Deficiency |
| -coele | Swelling or cavity | -pexy | Fixation |
| -desis | Bind together | -phasia | Speaking |
| -ectomy | Surgical removal | -pheresis | Removal |
| -emia | Blood condition | -plasia | Formation or development |
| -genic | Producing | -plasty | Surgical repair |
| -gram | A recording | -rhaphy | Surgical suture repair |
| -graph | A recording instrument | -scopy | Use of an instrument for viewing |
| -ia | Abnormal state | -stenosis | Narrowing |
| -itis | Inflammation | -stomy | Opening |
| -lysis | Destruction | -tomy | Cutting operation |
| -malacia | Softening | -version | Turning |
| -otomy | Surgical opening | | |

# Eureka! Putting them together

It should be apparent at this point that doctors and nurses are not the only ones who need to understand medical terminology. Your understanding the differences in terms is essential, as well, so that you can assign the correct codes.

After you understand prefixes and suffixes, you've got to make sense of the word as a whole. When you take the parts and assemble them, you have a medical term. Common terms assembled from the basic prefix/suffix combinations include the following:

✔ **Chondromalacia:** *Chondro-* refers to cartilage; *-malacia* means "softening," so *chondromalacia* means "softening of the cartilage."

✔ **Arthritis:** *Arthr-* refers to the joints; *-itis* means "inflammation," so *arthritis* means "inflammation of the joint."

✔ **Osteopenia:** *Osteo-* means "bone," and *-penia* means "deficiency." Therefore, *osteopenia* means "loss of bone."

✔ **Nephritis:** *Nephr-* refers to the kidneys, and *-itis* means "inflammation." Therefore, *nephritis* means "kidney infection."

✔ **Myalgia:** *My-* refers to muscles, and *-algia* means "pain." Therefore, *myalgia* means "pain the in muscles."

As you can see, the words can be mixed and matched as needed, and they take on different meanings as they are assembled. Adding to the potential confusion is the fact that many of the terms commonly used are quite similar and can seem deceptively close in meaning. To the untrained eye, they may actually seem to be the same. But the smallest of differences can make a big difference in reimbursement. The key to accurately charging the payer is a careful review of the record.

Here are a few examples of some similar-sounding terms that are actually different procedures. See whether you can spot the differences:

| *Term 1* | *Term 2* |
| --- | --- |
| *Arthrotomy* (surgery that is done through an open incision into a joint) | *Arthroscopy* (a surgical procedure performed by inserting a scope into a joint) |
| *Laparotomy* (surgery performed via an open incision into the abdominal cavity) | *Laparoscopy* (a surgical procedure performed by inserting a scope into the abdominal cavity) |
| *Tenodesis* (repair of a tendon that has been cut or torn) | *Tenolysis* (release of a tendon that is constricted by fibrosis or scar tissue) |

The same too-close-for-comfort issue is true of terms used to describe medical diagnosis (the topic of the next section); they may use similar terminology, but a minor distinction makes a big difference when you're coding. Here are some examples:

| *Term 1* | *Term 2* |
| --- | --- |
| *Hypertension* (high blood pressure) | *Hypotension* (low blood pressure) |
| *Bradycardia* (slow heartbeat) | *Tachycardia* (fast heartbeat) |
| *Angioplasty* (technique to treat blocked coronary arteries) | *Angiography* (technique to visualize and diagnose arterial disease) |

As the preceding examples show, you must read the record carefully to avoid costly errors.

# Understanding Medical Necessity

As I explain earlier, both diagnosis and procedures are linked to payment, so thoroughly understanding the diagnosis terms serves you well when you have to prove medical necessity to the payer.

Procedures and the reasons for performing them are at the heart of medical necessity. Put simply, the payer will absolutely, without fail, pay only for those procedures that are deemed medically necessary. For that reason, if you want the payer to approve payment (and you do), then you must make sure that the reason behind every procedure a medical professional performs is valid. For example, if the diagnosis code specifies a broken foot, the payer will pay only for the broken foot, not for a shoulder repair, even if both happened in the same accident. *The diagnosis must fit the procedure.* Seems pretty obvious, right?

It's not your responsibility as the coder to make up a payable diagnosis; it's your responsibility to *verify* that the diagnosis in the chart supports the procedure being billed. If you think the chart does not reflect the correct procedure, ask for clarification. Never make an assumption about what you think the physician meant to say. Take the time to follow up on any questions you have about the chart in question. Doing so saves you time and trouble later.

# Scrubbing In: Proving Medical Necessity for Surgical Procedures

When a physician performs a surgical procedure, no matter how simple or complicated, she makes a *preoperative diagnosis* based on test findings and examination. To confirm this preoperative diagnosis, the physician must be able to see inside the body cavity, either by cutting the patient open or by inserting a scope to see the inner workings. At that point, the doctor can make a *definitive diagnosis*.

You cannot code a surgical procedure from the preoperative diagnosis (also called a *preliminary diagnosis);* you can code the procedure only from the definitive diagnosis (also called the *post-operative findings).* Why? Because the physician can speculate about what she might find, but she can never really know until she performs the procedure.

You also need to examine the record closely to fully understand the approach the physician took and what she found. The approach lets you know whether the procedure was a traditional *open procedure*, one in which the patient's body is cut open, or a newer *endoscopic procedure*, in which a minimally invasive scope is used to perform a procedure inside the body. In the next sections, I explain the nuances of both types of approaches.

## Understanding endoscopic procedures

Many surgical procedures that you code are performed through the use of scopes. This type of procedure is generally referred to as *minimally invasive surgery*. Some operations can be completed entirely through a scope, while others are assisted by the use of a scope but still involve making an incision.

Some of the most common scope procedures are arthroscopic surgeries and laparoscopic procedures. The following sections have the details.

### Looking at arthroscopy

Arthroscopic surgery allows orthopedic surgeons to visualize, diagnose, and possibly treat injury or disease inside of a joint.

When a procedure is performed arthroscopically, the surgeon makes a minimum of two small incisions, called *portals,* into the joint. One incision is for visualization and the other is for the instruments, which are much smaller than traditional surgical instruments. Rather than directly view the surgical field (the area being operated on), the surgeon uses the scope to view the inside of the joint on a monitor. To make viewing the area easier, the joint is inflated with fluid, and additional portals may be created to view other areas within the joint.

Common arthroscopic procedures are performed on knees, shoulders, ankles, and hips. Small joints are also treated arthroscopically, but these procedures, such as carpal tunnel release, are less common and often are more time-consuming than traditional surgeries.

### Scope families

The American Medical Association (AMA) and American Academy of Orthopedic Surgeons (AAOS) categorize arthroscopic procedures into *scope families*. Simply put, scope families are procedures that go together.

Certain procedures are inherent to (automatically part of) other procedures that are performed. Because inherent procedures don't require additional time or skill by the surgeon, they're not eligible for additional reimbursement. Here's an example of a scope family procedure: arthroscopic chondroplasty inside the knee. The knee has three compartments: medial, lateral, and patello-femoral. Normally, the surgeon views all three compartments during a knee scope. Even if he shaves in each of the three areas, you can bill only one chondroplasty.

Different procedures that are performed in different compartments may be billable, depending on the documentation and the individual coding requirements for each compartment. The AMA and AAOS define what is separately billable and what is not. If you find yourself working in orthopedics, you need to learn what is and isn't considered a separate procedure. You can refer to the AMA website (www.ama-assn.org) and the AAOS website (www.aaos.org) for more information.

### Coding arthroscopic procedures

So how would you handle coding such a procedure? You've got to start with the documentation. The physician should document the surgery by compartment, clearly stating what he did in each compartment. The CPT book lists the different procedures that may have been performed. To be eligible for additional reimbursement, each procedure must have been fully documented as having been performed in different compartments. But be sure to check the edits because certain procedures — such as chondroplasty — are not to be separately reported unless they are the only procedures performed.

Sometimes a procedure is begun through a scope and then converted to an open procedure due to complications. When that happens, you code the open procedure only. Head to the section "Understanding open surgical procedures" for details on open surgical procedures.

## Defining laparoscopy

Laparoscopic surgery is a member of the endoscopy family, along with arthroscopy, except that laparoscopic surgery refers to the abdominal cavity (*laparo-* means "abdomen"); laparoscopic surgeries also include surgeries performed in the pelvic cavity. This type of procedure is another minimally invasive surgery that is sometimes called "Band-Aid surgery" because the incisions may have a suture, but they're often simply covered with a small bandage. Common laparoscopic procedures include gallbladder removal, appendectomies, ovarian cyst excisions, and numerous others.

### Understanding the procedure

Here's how laparoscopic surgeries work: Procedures are performed through a set of small portals in the abdomen. Similar to arthroscopic procedures, the physician views the interior of the abdomen on a monitor. During a laparoscopy, the abdomen is inflated with gas, which creates space that makes the areas easier to see and gives the surgeon more room to work.

At the beginning of the surgery, the scope is inserted through an incision near the navel, and the surgeon views inside the cavity to make sure that it's safe to proceed. If, during this inspection, the surgeon sees any medical reasons to stop the procedure (called *contra-indications*), the laparoscopic procedure is converted to a traditional open procedure (covered in the section "Understanding open surgical procedures"). Contra-indications include excessive inflammation or various other unknown risk factors.

If the surgeon feels that proceeding with the laparoscopy is safe, he creates additional portals for the specialized instruments needed to facilitate the necessary procedure(s).

Some procedures are *laparoscopically assisted*. An example is a hand-assisted laparoscopic surgery, in which the surgery is performed via a technique that uses a larger portal that allows for the insertion of a hand. This incision is larger than the traditional port but still smaller that a laparotomy incision. Surgeries performed laparoscopically normally require shorter recovery times and have fewer complications, compared to traditional open procedures.

### Families of laparoscopy

Laparoscopic procedures that go together are sometimes referred to as *families*. As explained in the earlier section "Scope families," procedures that are performed together as part of the necessary procedures may not be separately billable.

One common example in the laparoscopic world is a *diagnostic laparoscopy*. A physician may determine that the only way to really know what is going on with a patient is to take a look, using a diagnostic procedure. If that's all the doctor does, then the diagnostic procedure is billable. But if during this look-see, the surgeon sees something else — say an inflamed appendix — and removes it via laparoscopic appendectomy, then only the appendectomy can be billed.

## Understanding open surgical procedures

*Open surgery* refers to traditional surgical procedures, which involve an incision made by a surgeon. Obvious differences exist between endoscopic and open surgical procedures from a coding position. The distinction between -*otomy* versus -*oscopy* may seem minor, but it makes a big difference.

Being able to recognize such subtle differences between terms is why a solid knowledge of human anatomy and medical terminology is so important. Without it, you won't be able to tell one type of procedure from another.

### Coding the open surgical procedure

When you sit down to code an open procedure, you see the operative report, which includes the following:

✔ A heading that identifies the patient, the date and location of the surgery, the physician, and other demographic information.

The first step in abstracting the billable codes from the medical record of an open procedure is to identify which body part was treated and why. After you have identified that, you know which area of the CPT book to check to begin the process of coding.

✔ A preoperative, or preliminary, diagnosis, which is the diagnosis based on preoperative testing and pertinent physical findings observed by the physician during the examination

✔ The postoperative, or definitive, diagnosis, which is what the physician confirmed during the surgery.

✔ A summary or outline of the procedures performed.

Do not code procedures from the outline in the report! These headings are merely previews of what is to come. Regardless of what the heading says, for a procedure to be eligible for reimbursement, it must be documented in the body of the report.

✔ A full report containing the surgeon's description of everything that he did during the operation.

The documentation for the procedure should always be described in the body of the report. If the body of the report does not contain something that is mentioned in the heading, then the physician must correct the documentation before it can be reported. Remember the mantra of the medical coder: "If the doctor didn't say it, it wasn't done."

### Initiating a physician query

To get the missing information, you can initiate a physician query via a handwritten note (some facilities have a query form just for this purpose), or you can ask the surgeon directly for clarification if you work in an environment in which a direct query is possible. After you get an answer and if the record needs to be altered, the surgeon must dictate an addendum (add to the note), or he may dictate a corrected note.

When initiating a physician query, make sure that you don't lead the physician with regard to verbiage. Here are some examples of leading verbiage and more appropriate alternatives:

| *Leading* | *Non-leading* |
| --- | --- |
| Did the mass invade muscle tissue? | How deep was the mass? |
| Did you excise over one centimeter of the clavicle? | How much of the clavicle did you remove? |

Let the physician describe the work performed without putting words in his or her mouth.

### Understanding incidentals and unbundling

The surgeon may indicate that a certain procedure was extra or required additional time and skill on her part. If this extra work is well documented, it may support unbundling.

Unbundling procedures are affected by something called the National Correct Coding Initiative (NCCI) edits, which are the Medicare version of what is and isn't included or exclusive to other procedures. Most editing software programs are based on these edits. If the NCCI edits indicates that the procedures are bundled, then the physician must have documented that the procedures required additional skill and time before they can be billed separately.

For example, during a surgery, the surgeon has to make an incision, which is not billable. At the conclusion of the procedure, the surgeon needs to repair the incision, which is also not billable. Now, if the repair is more than what would be necessary to close the incision — say the surgeon has to rearrange tissue to improve the appearance of the scar — then the repair may be eligible for additional reimbursement, but the surgeon would have to document the additional work and the reason it was necessary. Otherwise, the procedure may be considered *incidental* and not separately billable.

As the coder, you're responsible for verifying which procedures are incidental and which ones are eligible to unbundle.

### Using billing modifiers

Certain modifiers are appropriate for surgical or diagnostic procedures; other modifiers are appropriate for claims submitted for reimbursement of office visits, referred to in the coding world as evaluation and management, or E&M, visits (covered in the next section). Here are the modifiers you're most likely to use:

- ✓ **Modifier 25:** You use this modifier when a procedure is performed on the same day that an E&M visit occurred. This modifier indicates that the procedure wasn't related to the E&M visit, and the provider feels that additional reimbursement is warranted.

- ✓ **Modifier 51:** This modifier indicates that multiple procedures have been submitted on one claim, and the appropriate discount may be applied.

   Most claims processing pay 100 percent of either negotiated rates or fee schedule reimbursement for the first procedure. Then additional procedures are paid at 50 percent of fee schedule, although some commercial payer contracts pay 25 percent of the third (or remaining) procedure(s) on each claim. Medicare pays 100 percent and 50 percent, regardless of the number of codes submitted. Other payer contracts may limit the number of procedures paid per encounter.

✔ **Modifier 59:** You use this magic modifier to indicate that a procedure being billed is normally included with another procedure or encounter but warrants separate consideration.

Correct reimbursement may depend upon using the appropriate modifier, and you're responsible for understanding which modifier to use when. But be careful. If you overuse or incorrectly use them, the provider can get into trouble.

# Connecting with the World of Evaluation and Management Codes

*Evaluation and management* (E&M) *codes* are the most commonly billed codes. These are the codes for every office visit and encounter a physician has with a patient, which typically involve non-invasive physician services.

When you use these codes, you find that your knowledge of medical terminology and medical necessity really comes into play because everything has a code! Here's a general list of the kinds of things that have their own E&M codes:

✔ Office visits by new patients

✔ Office visits by established patients

✔ Emergency room visits

✔ Observation visits (when the patient is in the hospital but not admitted because he's just being observed)

✔ Consultation visits (visits that have been requested by another physician, provider, or healthcare entity; read more about this in the section "Dealing with consultation visits")

Other codes include codes specific to hospitalized patients, codes for treating patients in nursing homes, critical care codes, and codes for assisted living/rest home visits.

The E&M visit may take place in a physician's office, nursing home, patient's home, hospital, emergency room, or clinic. *Note:* If the examination takes place during an office visit or a hospital visit, or if the patient has been referred for a specialized evaluation, the visit may technically be referred to as a *consultation,* which simply means that it's been requested by another physician or healthcare provider. Before you can bill a consultation, specific requirements must be met. I address those requirements later in this chapter.

## Looking at what happens during the run-of-the-mill E&M visit

As I explain earlier, E&M visits take place in multiple settings, but the basic structure is pretty much the same no matter the situation. Generally, you can break what happens during these visits down into three parts:

✔ **Gathering general information about the patient and the reason for the visit:** The first part of an E&M visit normally involves the physician asking the patient about the reason for the visit. The report you ultimately look at when you're coding includes the history of the present illness, the patient's personal history, the patient's family history, and information about the patient's social habits.

Patient history is a major component of an E&M code, and the more detail that is documented, the more easily the provider can justify higher reimbursement, if appropriate.

✔ **Conducting the physical examination:** The exam may involve a specific area of the body or several different areas. The more areas that the physician examines, the more detailed the examination. Again, examining multiple areas supports a higher level of reimbursement if the exam is thoroughly documented and appropriate for the patient's condition.

✔ **Determining the appropriate level of service:** The physician determines the appropriate level of service based on the presenting problem, the history and examination, and the amount of medical decision-making involved in the visit. This part of the visit greatly affects how you code the visit. The diagnosis, the plan for treatment, and the risk involved in treatment of the patient's illness are all factors you consider when choosing the appropriate level of decision-making for the CPT code to report the encounter. A more complex treatment plan or one that involves greater risk may justify a higher level of reimbursement.

The medical necessity of the presenting problem is the over-arching criterion for the level of service charged. If a patient has a cold, a doctor can take a full history and examine every single organ system and body part, but no medical necessity exists to charge a high level of visit because the patient just has a cold.

Read on for a more in-depth look at what takes place in an office and hospital setting and how it affects the way you go about your billing and coding business.

# Visiting the office

Office visits usually fall under the jurisdiction of E&M codes. Here are some things to pay attention to in order to ensure that the provider is reimbursed appropriately:

- **The reason for the visit:** This refers to the symptom(s) that caused the patient to schedule a visit with the physician. The physician documents the patient's initial complaint, along with his or her confirmation of the symptoms present.

- **The specific patient type (that is, whether the patient is new to the doctor or practice):** As the coder, you must verify whether the patient is new to the doctor or the practice, as well as the reason for the encounter. New patient visits have different CPT codes because an initial visit usually requires more of the physician's time and is therefore reimbursed at a higher rate. (New patients are those who are either completely new to the doctor or who have not been seen by the doctor or another one in the same practice for the past three years.)

- **Who is performing the service:** Some offices have nurse practitioners who see patients independently of the physician. Usually, these visits are reported under the practitioner's provider number, and depending upon the laws of individual states, normally a licensed physician must be present in the office suite when patients are being seen by any member of the staff.

The procedures or visit codes for physicians and practitioners are the same, but the payer often pays a different amount. Some payers want modifiers to indicate that the visit was with a member of the physician's clinical staff rather than the physician. It's your responsibility as the coder to be aware of individual payer requirements and bill appropriately as defined by the individual contracts. Some payers are finicky about paying for nurse practitioners or physician's' assistants, so make sure you learn the individual payer rules and keep the staff advised as necessary.

Sometimes a patient may visit the office, and the E&M code is not reportable. For example, if a patient comes in merely to receive a vaccination administered by a nurse, then the vaccination administration code may be the only reportable service. Billing for the drug may also be necessary, but you won't use an E&M code. (You can find the code for administering the vaccination in the Healthcare Common Procedure Coding System [HCPCS] book. HCPCS codes are used for various services — like administering vaccinations — drugs, and other medical equipment not found in the CPT book.)

Many offices use super-bills. These coding and billing shortcuts list the most common diagnoses and procedures performed by the practitioners. The physician checks the boxes to indicate what occurred during the visit. Make sure that you review the super-bill to ensure that all reported procedures are correctly documented in the record and that the indicated diagnosis supports medical necessity.

## Visiting the hospital

Choosing codes to report hospital visits by a physician can be a challenge for even the most experienced coders. Over-coding these visits can be an invitation for unwanted attention from payer audits, so you want to have a firm grasp of the different types of hospital codes, discussed in the following sections.

### Level-one, -two, and -three codes

Hospital visit codes have different levels:

- ✔ **Level-one codes (the patient is getting better):** This level of code is used to report the physician encounter that involves review of the patient's condition, both by examination and by the progress the hospital staff notes in the patient's chart. Normally, these visits are brief, and the level of decision-making is moderate, which means that, if the patient is recovering as anticipated, proceeding to the next step of treatment or recovery is okay.

- ✔ **Level-two codes (the patient isn't getting better):** With level-two codes, the patient isn't recovering as anticipated, so something else needs to be done. In this case, the physician discusses options with the patient and possibly issues revised orders for the staff; he may also order additional tests.

- ✔ **Level-three codes (the patient is declining fast):** This level of code is for the patients who have not responded to treatment or, worse, have continued to decline. Level-three visits require more of the physician's time and involve a higher level of decision-making, accompanied by a greater degree of risk for patient mortality.

Each level of coding comes with its own qualifying criteria. The level of medical decision-making is determined by the number of diagnoses present, the options for managing the illnesses, the amount or complexity of tests or data that the physician must review, and the level of risk to the patient for complications or death. So when a patient is initially admitted, you use specific codes to reflect that level of service. Then you use inpatient visit codes for services rendered during the patient's hospitalization.

If the patient is very ill, the higher-level codes may be justified; then as the patient's condition improves, you use lower-level codes.

In the event that the patient is critically ill and E&M codes are not appropriate, you use *critical care codes.* These codes are time-based and support a high level of reimbursement. Keep in mind, though, that they must be fully supported to be paid. So if you have inadequate documentation to support critical care, then the higher level of E&M code is probably a better choice.

### Inpatient and outpatient codes

Another consideration that defines the correct code choice is whether the patient is an inpatient or outpatient. Curiously, being in the hospital overnight does not necessarily mean that the patient is an inpatient. Here's the distinction:

- ✔ **Inpatient:** An *inpatient* is a person who has been officially admitted to the hospital under a physician's order. The patient remains an inpatient until the day before the day of discharge.

- ✔ **Outpatient:** A patient who comes through the emergency room and is being treated or who is undergoing tests but has not been admitted to the hospital is an *outpatient*, even if she spends the night.

Misrepresenting a patient's inpatient or outpatient status may lead to accusations of fraud, although sometimes the misrepresentation is unintentional. Documentation can be difficult to interpret when the patient status changes.

### Observation codes

You use observation service codes to bill for the physician's time when the patient is being seen at the hospital but the decision whether to admit has not been made. For example, a patient may come to the emergency room with chest pain, breathing difficulties, dangerously elevated blood pressure, or any number of symptoms, and that patient may spend one or two nights in the hospital. But if the physician has not written an order to admit the patient as an inpatient, it is an outpatient visit, and observation codes are the appropriate choice.

Always verify that a written order is part of the patient record, regardless of how often the physician sees the patient in the hospital setting. Without the written order, the visits are observations, or they may be consultation visits if the billing physician is seeing the patient at the request of another physician (see the later section "Dealing with consultation visits" for more info on coding those visits).

### Other hospital coding considerations

You must follow certain rules when reporting hospital visit codes. Some of these rules come from Medicare; others are specified contractually by the payer.

For example, if a provider visits a patient more than once in a calendar day, only one visit can be billed (this includes physicians from the same practice), but the level of reimbursement can be based on the documentation that supports the highest level. For example, if Dr. A visits the patient in the morning and his partner, Dr. B, stops by later in the day, you can bill only one visit to the payer if both doctors are in the same specialty. But if Dr. A is from the internal medicine office and Dr. B is from the cardiologist office, then they can both report the visit — as long as the visits are documented in the chart for medical necessity.

Similarly, some payers have limits on the number of physician visits they will pay for in one calendar day. If several specialists are simultaneously treating a patient, you need to know the payer guidelines with regard to number of visits, and each physician needs to document the reason for each visit.

The key point? Always choose the code based on the documentation provided. If the documentation is unclear, verify with the physician and ask for clarification — in writing — especially when you are coding different levels of service.

## Dealing with consultation visits

A consultation visit is simply a visit that's been requested by another physician, provider, or healthcare entity, such as a nurse practitioner, social worker, attorney, or even an insurance company.

With consultation visits, the most important thing for you to remember as a coder is to verify how the patient ended up seeing the physician. Most payers need to know that a visit to a consulting physician was medically necessary. In addition to detailing how the patient got connected to the consulting physician, the record must also document the request and reason for seeing the patient. The consulting physician must then send a report of his findings to the provider or healthcare entity that requested the consultation. The consulting physician may order tests or therapy as long as everything he does is included in a report back to the requesting physician or entity.

This game of Who Got Here and How isn't just confined to the clinical setting. It's also a big part of how you code what goes down in a hospital. When a physician puts on his consultation hat to see an inpatient, the request and reason for the consultation, as well as the consulting physician's findings, must be part of the patient record, which is shared in the case of an inpatient. When all this information is included in the patient's record, you can code such visits as consultation visits. (*Note:* There is an exception: If the consulting physician will be assuming care of the patient, you can't code the visit as a consulting visit. In that case, you use an inpatient code instead. Similarly, if all the treatment for a given problem is transferred to a consulting physician and he or she accepts the transfer before seeing the patient, the visit is not a consultation.)

Consultation visits are often time-consuming. If the physician invests a lot of time discussing test results, treatment options, and the like with the patient, a time-based consultation may be billable. When choosing one of these codes, the total time of the visit, along with the amount of time spent in counseling the patient, must be documented with the other required information. When documenting a time-based consultation visit, the record should indicate that at least half of the time reported was spent one-on-one with the patient, discussing test results, treatment options, and so on. A summary of the discussion should also be included in the record.

Be sure to verify whether a patient encounter is a consultation or a new patient visit. Consultation codes are the higher-paid E&M codes; therefore, solid documentation in the record is essential to support the additional reimbursement. If a consultation visit is missed, the reimbursement is lower than it should be. Conversely, if the patient is actually a new patient or a referred patient, then the service has been over-billed. (A referred patient differs from a patient sent for a consultation in that the referring physician does not make the request in writing, and the second physician will not necessarily send a report to the first physician.)

## Determining the level of billable service

The documentation that defines the services provided, the time spent with the patient, and the severity of the patient's condition determine the level of billable services. The sickness of the patient and the amount of work required by the physician is directly related to the level of reimbursement that is due.

The levels of service do not necessarily indicate the amount of time required to evaluate and treat the patient. The codes for those tasks — evaluating the patient's condition and deciding what steps are necessary to manage that condition — are the E&M codes; refer to the earlier section "Connecting with the World of Evaluation and Management Codes").

The appropriate level of service, however, *is* determined by how much work was required by the physician. As a rule, the sicker or more unstable the patient, the higher the level of service reported and coded — if the provider submits thorough documentation.

# Chapter 6

# Getting to Know the Payers

. . . . . . . . . . . . . . . . . . . . . . . . . . . . . . . . . . . . . . . . . . . . . . . . . . . . .

. . . . . . . . . . . . . . . . . . . . . . . . . . . . . . . . . . . . . . . . . . . . . . . . . . . . .

*A*fter you complete the coding, your work doesn't just go out into the void of space. It goes to the payer. A *payer* is the entity that reimburses the provider for services. Payers fall into three general categories: commercial payers (like insurance companies), government payers (like Medicare and Medicaid), and third-party administrators like American Insurance Administrators, Chickering Claims Administrators, or Healthnet, to name a few. Regardless of the payer type, every encounter between a provider and a patient is submitted to the payer as a claim.

To keep all these potential payers straight (as well as figure out who is supposed to pay you, how much, and when), you need to have the coding agility of a cheetah. Keep reading, and all will be revealed.

# The Man with the Plan: Commercial Insurance

The past 50 years have seen the healthcare industry develop into the behemoth it is today, and to no one's surprise, commercial insurance companies, which pay the majority of insurance claims, have become major cogs in the industry — so much so, in fact, that the patient without insurance may have difficulty securing affordable healthcare. Because commercial payers loom so largely in the big healthcare picture (commercial insurance administers the group health policies that most employers provide or supplement for their eligible employees), you've got to make their acquaintance because they'll show up frequently on your desk.

In the following sections, I outline who the different private carriers are and what you need to know about these plans to get the proper reimbursement.

## Buying higher levels of coverage

The more the individual contributes to the cost of the insurance, the better the coverage. Say, for example, that an employer offers different tiers of coverage:

✔ **Tier 1:** The employer offers first-tier coverage to the employee at no cost, but each doctor visit carries a $50 copay obligation, and the plan has a $2,000 major medical deductible. After the employee meets the deductible, the plan pays 70 percent of the covered expenses, and the employee is responsible for the other 30 percent. Employees who choose this option are gambling that they won't need to use the benefits too often.

✔ **Tier 2:** This plan may require the employee to contribute $100 per month toward his coverage, but the physician copay amounts are only $25, the annual deductible is $1,000, and the plan pays 80 percent of covered expenses. Employees who choose this option pay more for coverage, but that coverage is slightly more comprehensive.

✔ **Tier 3:** For this plan, the employee contributes $200 per month toward his coverage, but the copay is now $10 for a doctor visit. The deductible is waived, and the plan pays 90 percent of covered expenses. This is really good coverage, but the employee is paying for the additional benefits through the higher monthly contribution.

✔ **And so on:** Depending on what the employer offers, these tiers can be extended to include $0 copayment amounts and $0 deductible plans.

The decision is in the hands of the employee, and so is the gamble. Thus, by increasing up-front costs, the employee is betting that he'll need to use his insurance. On the flip side, by taking the plan offered at no cost, the employee is betting that he won't need to use his insurance. In all cases, the options available to the employee depend on what the employer offers.

## *Identifying the carriers*

The commercial insurance world revolves on an axis of variety. In fact, an insurance plan seems to exist for just about every situation, and providers see a variety of plans in their daily practices: preferred provider option plans; point of service plans; exclusive provider option plans; health maintenance organizations; high deductible plans; discount plans; and ultra-specific plans that provide only prescription coverage, vision coverage, or other specialized coverage. In the following sections, I take a look at some of the more common of these commercial plans.

The commercial insurance carrier is the company that writes the check to the provider, but the carrier may or may not be the one who prices the claim. Some carriers participate with payer *networks,* and the network prices the claims. Others may use third-party administrators (TPAs) to adjudicate, or price, their claims through their networks. To find out more about these entities, head to the later sections "Tuning in to networks" and "Choosing third-party administrators."

### Preferred provider organizations (PPOs)

A *preferred provider organization* (PPO) is a network of healthcare providers (doctors, hospitals, and so on) who have contracted with an insurer to provide healthcare services at reduced rates. The network contracts define reimbursement terms for all levels of service for the providers in the network.

Usually, patients with PPO plans are responsible for lower copayments and deductibles when they use a network provider, although they usually either pay higher premiums or have larger out-of-pocket costs than members of other plan types. On the plus side, PPO patients usually do not need a referral to see a specialist, but they may need to have certain procedures authorized in advanced.

### Health maintenance organizations (HMOs)

*Health maintenance organizations* (HMOs), which gained popularity in the 1970s, are organizations that contract with all types of providers (general practitioners, specialists, labs, hospitals, and so on) to create a patient service network from which the patient can choose or to whom the primary care physician can refer.

One benefit of the HMO to patients is lower-cost healthcare. They usually have lower premiums and little or no copay obligations. However, they must access all healthcare through an assigned *primary care physician* (PCP) who functions as a gatekeeper to control costs to the insurance company. Before patients can see a specialist, the PCP must refer them. Even with the required referral in hand, patients are still restricted to providers within the HMO's network.

Some HMOs have no out-of-network benefits. In this case — and depending on the provisions of the plan — the cost for the out-of-network services provided may fall on the healthcare provider or the patient. If a PPO-only provider sees an HMO patient, the PPO contract may force the provider to absorb the cost of patient treatment. If the provider has no contract with the company at all and sees an HMO patient, then the patient may be fully responsible for all costs. As the biller/coder, you'll see the results of these choices firsthand.

### Point of service plans (POS)

*Point of service* (POS) plans are a combination of PPO and HMO plans. A POS plan allows the patient to choose between PPO and HMO providers. POS members do not have to have a primary care physician, but they can if they want to. If they visit an HMO provider, they receive HMO benefits. If they choose to visit a PPO provider, they receive PPO benefits. POS patients usually have out-of-network benefits as well. Visiting a non–network provider increases the costs for the patients.

### Exclusive provider organization plans (EPOs)

*Exclusive provider organization* (EPO) plans are similar to HMO plans in that they typically require the patient to choose a primary care physician. They also require referrals if the services of a specialist are necessary, and the specialists must also be a network-contracted provider. The only exception is in the event of an emergency when a network provider is unavailable.

### High-deductible plans

The rising cost of healthcare has given birth to the high-deductible health plan. HMOs and PPOs started offering these plans in 2003. HMO and PPO deductibles are typically fairly low, but the premiums can become expensive. The high-deductible plans offer lower premiums but come with a high deductible. Deductibles in the $5,000 range are common. These plans are a smart choice for the young, healthy adult who rarely visits a doctor. But if that adult breaks a leg, the $5,000 adds up pretty darn quickly.

Some patients with high-deductible plans have health savings accounts (HSAs) or health reimbursement accounts (HRAs). HSAs are funded pre-tax by the insured; employers fund the HRAs. In addition, HRAs may or may not be handled by the same carrier; it depends on the group health plan provisions with the employer.

### Discount plans

Probably the plan with the fewest advantages for both patient and provider are discount plans. These plans require patients to pay a monthly fee, which gives them access to participating providers. The problem is that the patients pay for the services, supposedly at a discounted price.

These plans are not true health insurance, and plan members are usually shocked when they need to use their "insurance." It bears repeating, especially in this case: Always verify patient benefits in advance to protect the provider and the patient.

## Tuning in to networks

Some payers and providers participate in networks. A *network* is essentially a middleman that functions as an agent for commercial payers. The payers participate in networks who price claims for them. If a provider is contracted with a network and the insurance carrier is also part of that same network, then the network prices the claim, and the payer (carrier) pays the claim according to the network pricing.

## Wrapping your mind around COBRA

No insurance? No problem. At least, that's what you're supposed to think when you hear the word *COBRA*. Through COBRA (which stands for Consolidated Omnibus Budget Reconciliation Act), patients who leave their jobs (and the umbrella of the group plan) have the option to continue coverage so they don't go without some sort of healthcare option during their period of unemployment. COBRA applies to employers with 20 or more employees. Normal COBRA coverage is for 18 months, although certain qualifying conditions (such as a disability) may allow coverage for 36 months.

For the overage to stay in effect, the individual must pay COBRA premiums. If the individual makes monthly payments and a payment is late, a submitted claim may be rejected. If that happens, check with the patient to see

whether she paid the premium and then follow up with the payer to have the claim resubmitted. (Sometimes, the patient's check may have been received but not processed in time. Other times, if the payment is very late, a carrier may cancel the coverage.)

COBRA is not cheap. The price is typically based on the individual's current premium plus the portion paid by the employer. Throw in some administrative fees, and you can see why, when you're dealing with COBRA coding questions, the patients may seem a bit on edge. After all, they're already paying out the wazoo for extended coverage. The last thing they want to hear is that one of their procedures isn't covered. With COBRA, in particular, check and double check your coding work to avoid any unpleasant surprises for patients.

Some carriers participate with several different networks and have the claim priced according to the network that is most advantageous to them. For that reason, you want to know which networks your patients' plans access for pricing so that you can avoid unplanned write-offs. An easy way to find this information is to look at the insurance card to see whether it shows various network symbols, which represent a pricing network that the payer accesses for pricing claims.

A *write-off* is the part of the claim that neither the payer nor the patient pays. This particular part of the debt is forgiven. Most contracts define specific payment allowances per procedure. Regardless of the billed amount, the remaining dollar amount is contractually obligated to be written off by the billing provider.

## Choosing third-party administrators

*Third party administrators* (TPAs) are intermediaries who either operate as a network or access networks to price claims. TPAs often handle claims processing for employers who self-insure their employees rather than use a traditional group health plan. Also labor unions who offer coverage for members usually use TPA pricing.

The TPA functions as a network to price claims and serves the provider, the patient, and the employer by keeping healthcare costs under control. The reality is that most small companies are not in the healthcare business. They offer coverage to their employees but want to control the cost. By self-insuring — which means that the company actually pays the healthcare providers from a company account — the small company is, in theory, able to save money.

Here's how the cost savings is supposed to work: When a small company provides healthcare for its employees through a commercial carrier, the carrier prices the policy based on the health history and ages of the employees. Typically, a small group health plan costs a company about $450 per month per employee. If an employer chooses to self insure and uses a TPA, the employer pays a fee to be part of the network but then pays only the cost of the individual claims. The TPA negotiates the price through network pricing.

The downside of this arrangement is that, in the event of a catastrophe that affects several employees, the company could be in a dire financial situation. The success of using a TPA depends, in part, on playing the odds that something that lands everyone in the hospital won't happen.

Most providers view TPAs as run-of-the-mill network contracts, which they essentially are, although some TPA networks are funded by all parties. The provider may be responsible for paying a fee on adjudicated claims as part of the network agreement, and the insurer also pays a fee to participate in the network.

Understanding the difference between an insurer and a TPA is important, especially when claims don't process as expected, because the nature of the problem determines who you contact:

- ✔ If a TPA has incorrectly priced the claim, you need to address the issue through the TPA.
- ✔ If the payer didn't pay the claim according to the TPA pricing agreement, then you need to secure a copy of the claim adjudication sent to the payer and demand that the claim be reprocessed according to the pricing.

Check your checks and balances before you call — make sure you're barking up the right tree before you pursue a TPA claim.

# *Medicare: The Big Kahuna of Government Payers*

Beyond commercial payers (covered in the preceding sections) is good ol' Uncle Sam, who sponsors a variety of healthcare programs. The biggest is Medicare (for information on other government payers, like Medicaid, Tricare, and more, head to the section "Working with Other Government Payers."

Established in 1965 as part of the Social Security Act, Medicare provides insurance to people aged 65 and over, as well as to people with qualifying physical or mental disabilities. The program is financed by payroll taxes known as the Federal Insurance Contributions Act (FICA) tax. Both the employee and the employer pay this tax.

In the following sections, I outline the key things you need to know about Medicare.

The first Medicare beneficiary was former president Harry Truman. Actually, you don't really need to know this, but it's a fun fact anyway!

## *Examining Medicare, part by part*

As mentioned previously, four types of Medicare exist — Parts A through D — and each serves a particular purpose. The different types of Medicare and the fact that participation is automatic in some cases but not in others can lead to a lot of confusion with the plan's beneficiaries. Make sure you verify exactly which parts of Medicare are applicable to the patients you're dealing with before services are provided. I explain what you need to know in the following sections.

### *Medicare Part A*

Medicare Part A covers expenses for inpatient care in hospitals, skilled nursing facilities, hospice, and home healthcare.

Spending the night in a hospital does not necessarily mean that the visit is a Part A claim. The patient must have been admitted under physician orders to be an inpatient. Refer to Chapter 5 for information on the requirements that must be met to qualify as an inpatient.

### Medicare Part B

Medicare Part B helps pay for services deemed medically necessary. These services include physician services (including some preventative services like flu shots), outpatient visits, durable medical equipment, and home health services. Beneficiaries must enroll in Part B, and they pay a monthly premium. In addition, beneficiaries are responsible for paying an annual deductible and 20 percent co-insurance for Medicare-eligible services.

Some patients do not realize that Part B is optional, and they may mistakenly believe that they have it simply because they qualify for Medicare. Make sure you see the patient's Medicare card to verify Part B benefits.

Technically, enrollment in Part B is optional, but if you don't enroll when you're supposed to, you incur a penalty. If a person continues to work after age 65, enrollment may be deferred (that is, you can skip enrollment without penalty). Those who are no longer employed but fail to enroll have a 10 percent per year penalty added to the monthly premium. Eligible recipients who are still covered by group health coverage can delay enrollment in Part B until their group coverage ends. However, those individuals still need to be aware of the enrollment period that applies.

### Medicare Part C

Medicare Part C refers to replacement plans that some patients opt to enroll in. These replacement plans are offered by Medicare–approved private companies. Medicare replacement plans cover Part A and Part B services. Some plans also offer drug and vision coverage as well.

Medicare pays a fixed amount each month to companies that offer replacement plans, and in return, the companies agree to follow the rules set by Medicare for administration of the replacement plans. Each plan can charge out-of-pocket costs and can establish rules for plan use, such as requiring referrals to see specialists or requiring that the patient see only network providers.

Medicare-eligible patients who prefer private insurance enroll in Part C replacement plans. Some larger companies who historically have allowed retiring employees to stay on the company health plan are now offering Part C replacement plans to eligible enrollees. Some companies with employees who are Medicare eligible offer these employees Part C plans as well.

When coding for services provided to these patients, make sure that you verify coverage and plan restrictions prior to any encounter. Commercial plans follow commercial contract obligations, and the Medicare plans have to follow Medicare payment guidelines unless the commercial contract contains a Medicare Part C reimbursement clause that obligates the payer to a specific payment or fee schedule different than standard Medicare.

You can avert unnecessary appeals by verifying Part C enrollment early in your coding process. Verification of Medicare patients is fairly simple. Some of the Medicare contractors have websites that let providers check patient benefits. Others have *interactive voice response* (IVR) telephone systems that providers can call to check patient coverage.

### Medicare Part D

Medicare Part D is Medicare's prescription drug plan. Medicare-approved companies run these plans. To participate, qualifying individuals must enroll in a plan and adhere to plan restrictions.

Part D normally does not affect healthcare providers or their staff. But some patients can be confused and think they've enrolled in a Medicare supplement (explained in the next section) when what they have is a Part D plan to cover prescription drugs. In these situations, you may find yourself explaining to the patient the difference between another major medical plan and a Medicare supplement plan.

## Looking at Medicare supplement policies

Medicare supplement policies cover the charges that Medicare doesn't pay. Normally, Medicare pays 80 percent of allowed expenses after the participants meet the annual deductible. Many patients enroll in secondary coverage to make up the difference. For example, these plan may cover the annual Medicare deductible and the 20 percent co-insurance left over by Medicare. These supplements don't cover expenses that Medicare doesn't approve, however.

A true Medicare supplement serves as a gap coverage to pay what Medicare approves but doesn't pay. Medicare patients do not usually benefit by carrying a second major medical plan such as those discussed earlier in the chapter, and they are surprised when faced with unplanned medical expenses. Your best bet is to verify secondary coverage in addition to Medicare eligibility prior to any patient encounter. The question you need to ask as a coder is "Does this secondary plan cover what Medicare approves but does not pay?"

## Other things to know about coding and processing Medicare claims

It probably comes as no surprise to you that coding and processing Medicare claims can get pretty confusing. In the following sections, I give you the lowdown.

# Crossing over

Some Medicare supplement policies accept claims directly from Medicare, a practice known as *cross-over claim submission.* Patients with these plans need to let Medicare know that they have a Medicare supplement plan, the details of that plan, and the effective date. Then, after Medicare processes a claim, it sends the claim directly to the secondary payer, and the provider is paid in a more timely fashion. Ta-da! Cross-over claim at work.

Some other supplemental Medicare carriers claims will cross over, but they are not automatic. These are known as *Medigap policies.* To get Medigap policies to cross over, a provider needs to enter the policy holder, policy number, and name of the plan on the HCFA-1500 or UB-04 along with the carrier's assigned Medigap number.

Secondary complementary claims or Medigap claims don't automatically cross over to the secondary carrier if the claim is totally denied, a duplicate claim, an adjustment claim, a claim that has been reimbursed by Medicare at 100 percent, a claim that is submitted to Medicare outside the eligibility dates, or a claim for a provider who doesn't participate with Medicare. (*Note:* When the cross-over action is automatic, you don't have a chance to correct an error on a claim.)

### The coding criteria

Medicare strictly adheres to the established National Correct Coding Initiative (NCCI) edits, along with procedure/medical necessity protocol. In addition, its claims processing system is highly refined. Any claim that is submitted with errors or without the correct information does not process, period. For detailed information on how to submit an error-free claim, head to Chapter 12.

### Rules regarding payouts

Congress legislates how Medicare claims are paid out to providers. Here's what you need to know:

- ✔ The payer has what is called a *payment floor,* a set length of time to complete and process claims. When the service dates have been released for payment, then Medicare pays.

- ✔ Medicare prefers to pay with the electronic fund transfer (EFT), which helps solidify Medicare's reputation as a good payer who pays most claims without incident if they are submitted correctly.

Make sure you're familiar with the Medicare contractor's claim submission preference and submit claims accordingly because Medicare is not going to adapt to provider needs; the provider does all of the adapting!

### The role of MACs, LCDs, and ABNs

Through Medicare, the Centers for Medicare & Medicaid Services (CMS) sets the rules for the country, but Medicare claims processing happens in regional areas. CMS contracts with private companies, called Medicare Administrative Contractors (MACs), to process Medicare claims. MACs have replaced the former system of fiscal intermediaries (who processed Part A claims) and the local carriers (who processed Part B claims).

As Medicare contractors, MACs may develop or adopt policies in the following circumstances:

- ✔ When no national coverage determination regarding a specific procedure exists. (Basically, *national coverage determination* refers to a nationwide determination of whether Medicare will pay for a service or not.)

- ✔ When a need to further define a national coverage determination exists.

When a local contractor adopts such a policy, it is known as an LCD, or *local coverage determination.* The Medicare Program Integrity Manual contains the guidelines for LCD policy development. You can check it out at www.cms.gov/manuals.

Most coding software can identify local coverage restrictions. Use it whenever possible. The CPT books have a symbol next to procedures that may have local coverage restrictions that you need to review prior to submitting a claim.

If a service or diagnosis is not covered by CMS, the MAC can't agree to cover it. A provider who furnishes a service that Medicare probably won't cover can ask the patient to sign an *advanced beneficiary notice* (ABN). By signing an ABN, the patient agrees to be financially responsible for the service if Medicare denies payment. If the provider doesn't offer the ABN or the patient doesn't sign the notice before services are rendered, the patient doesn't have to pay for that service.

As a coder, you must be familiar with the local coverage policies of your Medicare contractor so that you can submit claims correctly. If a service is provided that is processed incorrectly, a solid knowledge of payment rules can help you resolve the issue.

# Working with Other Government Payers

Medicare may be the biggest but it isn't the only government payer. Some of those with the greatest presence are Tricare (for military personnel and their dependents), the Department of Labor (for injured federal workers), and Medicaid (for the poor). Each has its own individual billing requirements. Keep reading for the details.

# Medicaid

Medicaid, like Medicare, was created by the 1965 Social Security Act. Its purpose is to assist low-income people pay for part or all of their medical bills. Medicaid is federally governed but locally administered.

Medicaid falls into two general types:

- ✔ **Community Medicaid**, which assists eligible beneficiaries who have no (or very little) medical coverage
- ✔ **Medicaid nursing home coverage**, which pays for nursing home costs for eligible recipients. These beneficiaries pay most of their income toward nursing home costs.

In the next sections, I explain how Medicaid is funded and administered, who qualifies for the program, and what you as a coder need to pay attention to when dealing with Medicaid claims.

## Administering and funding Medicaid

The Medicaid program is administered through the U.S. Department of Health & Human Services (HHS) through CMS. Each state is responsible for implementing its own Medicaid program, although CMS establishes the program requirements and monitors the programs to ensure compliance with federal policies and procedures. Participation in Medicaid is voluntary, yet every state participates and is required to follow the CMS protocol for service quality and eligibility standards.

Federal regulations define the minimum medical services that must be provided to a Medicaid patient. These services include inpatient hospital treatment, pregnancy and prenatal care, and surgical dental services. Individual states may provide additional care when funding allows.

Several states combine Medicaid programs with other insurance programs, such as those directed at children. Some states use private health insurance companies to administer their Medicaid programs. These providers are essentially HMOs that contract with the state Medicaid department to provide services for an agreed-upon price. Other states work directly with the service providers.

The federal government and the states share funding for Medicaid. Some states receive additional funding assistance from counties.

### Program eligibility

Program eligibility is determined primarily by income and access to financial resources. For example, having limited assets is a primary requirement for eligibility. In addition to demonstrating poverty, though, eligible recipients must fall into another eligibility category as defined by CMS. These categories include age, pregnancy, disability, blindness, and status as a U.S citizen or lawfully admitted immigrant. Special exceptions are made for those living in nursing homes and disabled children residing at home. A child, for example, may be eligible regardless of the eligibility of the parents or guardians.

Individuals who meet other eligibility requirements but don't meet the income or asset requirement have a *spend down,* in which they reduce their assets so that they can qualify for Medicaid. Federal guidelines permit spend downs, but not all state programs allow them. Patients having a spend down pay for healthcare costs out of their own pockets, using their own resources, until their asset levels fall enough to qualify for Medicaid coverage.

### Things to watch for when coding Medicaid claims

When billing for a Medicaid patient, you need to research the state's Medicaid billing requirements. Some carriers want certain modifiers; others don't. Verifying a patient's eligibility status with Medicaid is usually difficult. Generally, you can only verify whether the patient has it and whether a referral is needed. The spend down, if there is one, can't be determined until after the claim has been submitted for consideration.

Many Medicaid policies are secondary to Medicare. If the patient has kept Medicare advised, the claim usually crosses directly from Medicare to be processed. Unlike other secondary payers, however, Medicaid usually pays per its fee schedule, regardless of what the primary payer pays. For example, if a primary commercial insurance contract obligates a claim to pay $1,000, but the Medicaid fee schedule obligates the same procedure to pay $500, Medicaid pays $500, and the issue is closed.

# Tricare (Department of Defense)

Tricare, funded by the U.S. Department of Defense, is the healthcare system used by active military personnel and their dependents.

Different Tricare programs address the needs of specific segments of the military:

✔ **Tricare Standard:** Active duty military, retired active duty military, reserve military retirees, and eligible family members use Tricare Standard. These members can use any civilian healthcare provider and usually have a co-insurance responsibility and a deductible.

✔ **Tricare Prime:** Tricare Prime serves the same segment of the military population that Tricare Standard does, except that Tricare Prime is more restrictive. Tricare Prime patients are allowed to seek treatment only from network providers. All active military are required to enroll in Tricare Prime, but for eligible dependents, it's a less expensive option.

✔ **Tricare for Life:** Tricare for Life is essentially a Medicare supplement available to retirees who were formally Tricare members that became Medicare eligible. (Go to "Looking at Medicare supplement policies" for info.)

To put it in insurance terms, think of Tricare Standard as the military equivalent of a PPO. Tricare Prime, which is more restrictive, is the equivalent of an HMO. Think of Tricare for Life as a Medicare supplement policy.

In the United States, Tricare benefits are administered through regional contractors known as Tricare North, Tricare South, and Tricare West. Overseas claims are processed through the Tricare Overseas Program.

Tricare follows the same claim editing programs that Medicare uses, and it pays according to Tricare fee schedules. A provider who treats a Tricare patient can expect the claim to process per the appropriate fee schedule; in return, Tricare trusts the provider to accept the fee schedule pricing and not to send the balance to the patient to pay (a practice called *balance billing*), regardless of a network contract.

The fee schedules are updated regularly; you can access them through the Tricare web portals.

## CHAMPUS VA (Department of Veterans Affairs)

CHAMPUS (Civilian Health and Medical Program of the Uniformed Services) VA patients are those who are not eligible for Tricare: spouses or dependents of veterans disabled in the line of duty and surviving spouses of veterans who had been disabled or died from a service-connected disability. (Occasionally a surviving spouse or child of a military member killed in the line of duty may have CHAMPUS VA, but normally they are eligible for Tricare.)

CHAMPUS VA plans are always secondary when another payer exists. When CHAMPUS VA is the primary payer, it functions mostly like an HMO. Always verify patient coverage prior to any scheduled encounters to secure any necessary referrals or prior authorization for treatment.

In prior years, both active and retired military beneficiaries and their dependents were treated exclusively at military facilities. Due to budget restrictions, the Department of Defense started to contract with civilian providers for their members' healthcare needs. This program was originally known as CHAMPUS. Later, CHAMPUS became CHAMPUS VA, which is now funded by the Veterans Administration.

# Office of Workers' Compensation Programs (Department of Labor)

The U.S. Department of Labor's Office of Workers' Compensation Programs (OWCP) administers disability compensation programs to injured federal workers or those who acquire an occupational disease. Workers' Compensation claims can be a bit tricky. Here's what you need to do when you work with these types of claims:

- ✔ **Follow the filing requirements established by the Department of Labor (DOL).** First, providers must enroll, after which, they are assigned a DOL provider number. Second, DOL claims always require prior authorization for each procedure (even though pre-authorization doesn't necessarily guarantee reimbursement), and each procedure must be supported by the approved condition being treated (medical necessity). Only the approved diagnosis for the patient's treatable condition is accepted on these claims.

- ✔ **Prior to treating a patient who tells you he has been injured on the job, verify Workers' Compensation claim information with the patient's employer or the Workers' Comp carrier if you have that information.** Verify the claim number, date of injury, and the body part approved for treatment. Also get the adjuster's name and contact information and verify the submission address for the claims.

- ✔ **Verify the approved diagnosis code.** The Workers' Compensation carrier has one or two approved diagnoses that must be used for all claims submissions. The treating physician must know what these approved diagnoses are so that the treatment administered is supported by medical necessity. If you vary from these diagnoses, your provider won't be paid.

✔ **Make sure all reportable procedures have been pre-authorized.** All OWCP claims need to be pre-authorized. Although pre-certification does not guarantee payment, failure to pre-certify guarantees no payment.

✔ **Include the medical records with the claims.** Any treatment to be paid for must be a result of the injury. If the Workers' Compensation patient with the injured shoulder also has bronchitis, for example, the bronchitis is probably not an approved diagnosis.

✔ **Provide regular follow up.** As with any other government program, you must navigate through the maze associated with each individual claim.

Similar to other federal insurance programs, OWCP processes claims based on a fee schedule. The DOL fee schedule, in addition to CCI edits, are used to process DOL claims. You can access the DOL fee schedule via a link on its website (`http://owcp.dol.acs-inc.com`). To access this portal, the provider must register and request a login. Also, payments for DOL claims are made via electronic fund transfer (EFT). Prior to submitting any DOL claims, part of the enrollment process is to also enroll for the EFTs.

With Workers' Comp claims, not only are you billing and coding for the benefit of the provider or payer, but you are also coding something that will affect whether someone receives proper compensation for a possible at-work injury. A lot is at stake for everyone involved. For that reason, you've got to be on top of your coding game, even more so than usual. For specific information regarding OWCP claims, go to the Department of Labor's website (`www.dol.gov`).

The DOL has the three divisions:

✔ **Federal Employees' Compensation Act (FECA):** This covers the majority of DOL claims.

✔ **Division of Coal Mine Workers' Compensation (DCMWC):** This division is dedicated to coal workers' claims.

✔ **Division of Energy Employees Occupational Illness Compensation (DEEOIC):** This division is dedicated to the claims involving federal employees of the Division of Energy.

# Part III

# Keys to Becoming a Professional: Getting Certified

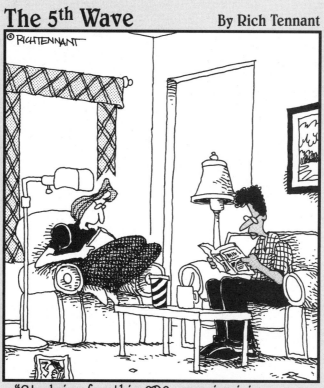

The 5th Wave                    By Rich Tennant

"Studying for this CPC exam is giving me a 307.81 in the gluteus maximus."

# In this part . . .

In billing and coding, being certifiable is a good thing. No, I'm not talking about your sanity (or lack thereof). Certification is at the root of everything you need to do to build a billing and coding career, and the best way to prepare for your certification exams is to complete a training program.

In this part, I tell you about the different kinds of certifications and describe how to find a reputable training program. And because being the best in your field means not resting on your laurels, I also tell you how you can bolster your credentials through specialty certifications and continuing ed.

# Chapter 7

# Your Basic Certification Options, Courtesy of the AAPC and AHIMA

. . . . . . . . . . . . . . . . . . . . . . . . . . . . . . . . . . . . . . . . . . . . .

### In This Chapter

▶ Getting to know the two main credentialing organizations: the AAPC and AHIMA

▶ Identifying the type of certification that best fits your career goals

▶ Knowing what to expect for each type of certification exam

. . . . . . . . . . . . . . . . . . . . . . . . . . . . . . . . . . . . . . . . . . . . .

*F*or success as a medical biller and coder, you've got to be certified by a trusted credentialing organization like the AAPC or AHIMA. Each organization is different and has its own unique credentialing requirements.

Each type of certification offered by these organizations has different benefits, depending on what you want to do in your billing and coding career. Some gear you up for work in a physician's office; others prepare you for the hospital environment. Plus, the type of certification you decide to pursue affects what kind of training program you end up in, because many of the training programs are specifically geared to particular types of certification exams. For those reasons, you need to give thought to what you want to do in your career before you make that all-important certification choice.

In this chapter, I introduce you to these credentialing organizations, explain the basic certifications they offer, and give you a general idea of what to expect on their certification exams. (You can read about specialty certifications in Chapter 10.)

# Introducing the Two Main Credentialing Organizations: The AAPC and AHIMA

The AAPC (formerly the American Academy of Professional Coders) and the American Health Information Management Association (AHIMA) are the two primary credentialing organizations. AHIMA certification covers coding in hospitals, and AAPC certification covers everybody else.

The AAPC was founded in 1988 with two goals: providing education and professional certification to medical coders working in physicians' offices and setting a higher standard of coding by adhering to accepted standards. AHIMA's certifications are primarily directed at coders working in hospitals. Founded in 1928, AHIMA's original goal was to improve the quality of medical records; today it continues to strive for excellence in medical record integrity with the evolution of electronic medical records. Both the AAPC and AHIMA offer educational resources and programs including certifications.

Prior to applying for membership in either organization and registering to take a certification exam, research each one to see which best fits your need and your budget. You also may want to find out when and where the local chapter meets and attend a meeting or two just to get the feel of the organization's culture. And feel free to press some flesh and talk people up: Both organizations offer network and mentoring opportunities.

## Going with the AAPC . . .

The AAPC is widely recognized for credentialing both physician- and hospital-based coders and is expanding to offer physician training services to practices as well as a credential for healthcare attorneys and IT staff. Its training programs are offered throughout the United States. The organization also offers access to continuing education opportunities and a job database. In addition to regional conferences, the AAPC has a national convention every year, where you can find both educational and networking opportunities. (The regional conferences offer the same opportunities and are usually more economical.)

## Choosing AHIMA instead

AHIMA is highly respected in the area of hospital and physician coders. The organization offers a variety of training programs, has an annual convention, and conducts workshops lasting several days in a variety of locales. If you choose to be credentialed by the AHIMA, you'll have access to training and networking opportunities throughout your career.

Although it offers entry-level credentials, AHIMA doesn't offer apprentice-level certifications as AAPC does. AHIMA certifications are intended for those already intimately familiar with coding.

## *Be a joiner: The benefits of membership*

In today's world of privacy and compliance concerns, certification is the industry standard. Because certification shows that you are proficient in your area and are committed to quality healthcare by disseminating quality information, it's one of the first qualifications that employers look for when they review you as a potential candidate, and it's an asset when you're negotiating a salary. In addition, the majority of billing companies have contracts with their clients that obligate them to hire only certified coders.

As a member of one of the two main credentialing organizations —AHIMA or AAPC — you're privy to different professional goodies. Both organizations provide numerous networking opportunities. In addiiton, AAPC members receive discounts on certification tests, preparation materials, workshop fees, and numerous other products. They also are automatically subscribed to the association's monthly publication, *The Coding Edge,* which keeps members up to date on changes and offers continuing education units (you can read more about those in the section "Building on Your Cred with Continuing Education"). Similarly, AHIMA members enjoy membership perks such as access to professional publications, discounts on books, and other training opportunities open to members only.

## Figuring your return on investment

It really does pay to be a certified medical biller/coder, no matter what designation you choose to pursue. Surveys conducted by the AAPC indicate that coder salaries have continued to increase despite economic downturns. One possible reason for this is that getting payers to pay claims is becoming increasingly difficult. Because reimbursement is code-based, providers are even more dependent on hiring people with strong billing and coding expertise than ever before. As an experienced coder, you practically pay for your own salary with the money you save your employers and through your ability to abstract all billable procedures from the medical record.

Another bonus of certification is that you have access to multiple career paths and a greater salary potential. The more certifications you have, the more employment options are open to you. Many coders who responded to the AAPC survey indicated that their duties involved more than just coding, and many of them took on and got paid for more responsibility in their workplaces. For example, a solid knowledge of coding is a bonus for billing managers, account receivable representatives, and medical practice managers. And those titles equal more money in your pocket!

Trust me when I say that getting the proper certification is money in the bank for you. Doing so ensures that you have the proof of abilities, which will, in turn, get you the job you really want. And if you want to tack on even more certifications, you can do that. In Chapter 10, I give you the 411 on the myriad specialty certifications you can add to make yourself even more marketable.

## *Joining one or both: The pros and cons of multiple membership*

You may be wondering, since certification offers so many benefits, whether you can compound your advantages by having more than one certification. Very possibly. But before you begin signing up for every certification possible, consider the pros and cons of having multiple certifications:

- ✔ **Potentially higher salary:** Theoretically, the more certification levels you achieve, the higher the salary you can expect. In reality, *experience* plus certification improves your marketability tenfold. In other words, don't go certification crazy without earning some real-world experience to go along with all of those acronyms.

- ✔ **More access to networking opportunities:** Multiple memberships mean increased network opportunity. If you attend local chapter meetings and become an involved member, when a job becomes available, someone with influence may suggest you or serve as a reference.

- ✔ **Increasing costs to achieve multiple certifications:** One big disadvantage of multiple certifications is cost. The initial cost of taking the test(s) can be a drain on your personal finances. In addition, each certification requires a certain number of continuing education units (CEUs) within your chosen specialty. (Chapter 10 has info about continuing ed.)

- ✔ **Higher membership dues:** The other disadvantage is the cost of membership. Some employers may reimburse your dues or other costs, but don't count on it, especially in the beginning.

# *Looking at the Basic Certifications*

As I explain in the earlier sections, if you want to get ahead as a medical biller and coder, certification is a must. The trick is knowing which certification organization is most appropriate for you and whether you'd be best served by having multiple certifications.

AAPC and AHIMA are the most well-known (read: trusted) organizations, so their certifications likely open more doors. Choosing the right certification depends on your experience and eligibility to take the exam(s). In the following sections, I discuss what each organization offers and other things you need to think about. (***Note:*** Both organizations also offer specialty certifications. You can read about those in Chapter 10.)

# The AAPC and its basic certifications: CPC, CPC-H, CPC-P

Starting at the top of the heap, you'll want to think about AAPC certification and what it can or can't do for your coding career. The basic certification level for the AACP is the CPC certification. This certification indicates proficiency in reading a medical chart and abstracting the correct diagnosis codes, procedural codes, and supply codes. It's the certification level most members first attain.

As a CPC-certified coder, your best fit is in a physician's office, billing office, or certain other outpatient environments, where you're expected to have a thorough understanding of anatomy and medical terminology and be able to apply procedural codes and the supporting diagnosis codes. Other basic CPC certifications include CPC-H and CPC-P. You can see a quick description of all these certifications in Table 7-1.

| Table 7-1 | Basic AAPC Certifications |
|---|---|
| *Certification* | *Related Skills and Competencies* |
| Certified Professional Coder (CPC) | Proficiency in reading medical charts and assigning correct diagnosis (ICD-9) codes, procedure codes (CPT), and supply codes (HCPCS) |
| Certified Professional Coder-Hospital (CPC-H) | Proficiency in assigning accurate codes for diagnosis, procedures, and services performed in an outpatient setting; understanding compliance and outpatient grouping systems; and completing a UB-04, the billing form used for facility claims, with appropriate modifiers |
| Certified Professional Coder-Payer (CPC-P) | Proficiency in understanding the claim adjudication process; possessing basic knowledge of coding-related payer processes, including the relationship between coding and payment |

The AAPC has stringent eligibility requirements for full certification. If you have two years of coding experience before you take the exam, you'll be fully certified upon passing. If you don't have experience in coding prior to sitting for the exam for any of these certifications, you'll earn an apprentice status: CPC-A, CPC-H-A, or CPC-P-A. After you complete your apprenticeship, you can request that the A be removed by following either of the following processes:

✔ **Send a request, along with two letters verifying that you've had at least two years of experience using the coding books.** At least one letter should be on letterhead from your employer, and the other may be from a co-worker. Both letters must be signed and should outline your coding experience and amount of time in that capacity. Alternatively, to speed the process up, your references can fill out the Apprentice Removal Template available on the AAPC website. However, letterhead and signatures are still required.

✔ **Prove that you have completed at least 80 hours of coding education and have completed one year of on-the-job experience using CPT, ICD, and HCPCS codes.** This can be a certificate of course completion, a letter from your instructor on school letterhead, or a transcript that states that you have completed a minimum of 80 hours of classroom training. If you choose this option, you also must provide one letter on letterhead that has been signed by your employer that verifies that you have completed one year of on-the-job experience.

## AHIMA and its basic certifications: CCA, CCS, CCS-P

Although AHIMA certification is most desirable for hospital-based coders, this certification is also accepted in physician practices or practice management companies.

Here are the basic certificaitons offered by AHIMA:

✔ **Certified Coding Associate (CCA):** This certifies that the coder has demonstrated proficiency in inpatient and outpatient hospital-based coding. It's a nice overall certification that prepares you for multiple environments.

Although the CCA exhibits competency in both clinical and hospital settings, it doesn't show that you have a mastery of either. If you want to go for the higher tier of certification, go with the CCS or its physician-specific counterpart, the CCS-P, which I explain in the next two items in this list.

✔ **Correct Coding Specialist (CCS):** This is the main certification offered by AHIMA. It indicates that you have competency in hospital coding, and it requires a higher level of expertise in diagnosis and procedural coding than the CCA certification does, because as a CCS, you are able to abstract codes from patient records.

People who attain this certification are also experts in both CPT and ICD coding systems. And just like CPC-certified coders, the CCS possesses a strong knowledge of medical terminology and human anatomy. The CCS curriculum also contains instruction in the disease process and pharmacology. Whew! That's a lot to take in. But, hey, if working in a big hospital is your bag, then you're going to interface with all kinds of people and situations. The CCS helps you get ready for all of it.

✔ **Correct Coding Specialist-Physician Based (CCS-P):** This certification indicates that you specialize in physician settings, such as physician offices, and are responsible for assigning ICD-9 diagnosis and CPT procedure codes based on patient records. You have thorough knowledge of health information and are dedicated to data quality and integrity because data submitted to insurance companies determines the level of reimbursement to which the physician is entitled.

# Choosing the Certification That's Right for You

Deciding which type of certification best fits your career goals is really a two-step process. Think about these two factors when you are selecting a certification type:

✔ **The type of training program you want:** How much time can you dedicate to a training program? What's your budget? What sort of curriculum interests you?

✔ **Your long-term career goals:** What kind of medical billing and coding job do you ultimately want to do? In what sort of facility do you want to work? How do you want to spend your time each day?

Your answers to those questions can help you choose what kind of certification will most benefit your long-term goals and short-term educational needs. Read on for more details.

The thing you need to remember about AAPC and AHIMA when choosing a type of certification is that each organization's certifications are designed to help you fit in the career niche of your choice. (*Note:* You can attain several other types of certification, including numerous specialty certifications you can add on top of your primary certification. To find out about these certifications, go to Chapter 10.)

## Looking at the educational requirements

Some certifications require you to earn a four-year degree prior to taking the exam, while others require little more than a short-term program under your belt. Both AHIMA and AAPC recommend that you complete some type of accredited training program. These accredited programs provide the education and training you need to work in the healthcare industry and to pass that exam. Your other pre-test training options include vocational training schools and online programs.

Most programs offer training in subjects like human anatomy and physiology; medical terminology and documentation; medical coding, including proper use of modifiers; medical billing; and more.

Each training option has its pros and cons, but the most important qualities to look for in a training program are accreditation and the expertise of the instructors teaching the classes. Head to Chapter 8 for a complete discussion of training programs, the degrees offered, and how to choose a program that's right for you.

## Prioritizing your career needs

Although you can't predict the future, you can put some thought into your long-term career needs when you're thinking about the type of training program you want. The last thing you want is to get stuck in a program that prepares you for a certification exam that doesn't match up with how you want to spend the rest of your career. As you talk your way through this decision, consider these factors:

- ✔ Where you plan to seek employment (hospital, physician's office, and so on)

- ✔ The kind of job you want to do (coding, medical billing, charge posting, or accounts receivable follow-up)

    Coders tend to be introverted and detail-focused and are happiest working quietly on their own. If that appeals to your personality, then coding may be a good choice, as would other positions that tend to attract people with those same qualities, like medical billing or charge posting. If you're more social, you may be happier in accounts receivable follow-up because this position requires constant interaction with others (payers).

- ✔ The type of certification potential employers might prefer

- ✔ The availability, quality, and cost of the training programs in your area

## Seeing what employers in your area want

Where you want to work and what kind of job you want to do will probably carry the most weight in your decision-making process. After all, you want to make yourself the most marketable candidate for the jobs you want most. Try these tips for tracking the ins and outs of potential employers and, by extension, the certifications they require:

- ✔ Check with local employment recruiters and see what type of credentials their clients prefer.

- ✔ Take note of the credentials displayed in local medical offices that you visit.

- ✔ Look through the local job listings and see what kinds of certifications are mentioned in jobs that appeal to you.

- ✔ If you have your heart set on working for a particular company, find out what kind of coders they prefer. If the local hospital only uses AHIMA certified coders and records clerks, then you want to find an AHIMA-accredited program and take an AHIMA exam. On the other hand, if that same hospital employs both AAPC- and AHIMA-certified professionals, then you need to find the program that best prepares you to take the exam that'll give you the best chance to score a job.

# Examining the Exams: A Quick Review of the Main Tests

After you've given thought to what sort of medical billing and coding career you want and have an understanding of what the standard educational path for a medical biller and coder is, you're ready to research the main certification exam options. And — no big surprise here — you can start by getting to know the exams offered by the AAPC and AHIMA: the Certified Professional Coder (CPC) exam, offered by AAPC, and the Correct Coding Specialist (CCS) exam and the Certified Coding Associate (CCA) exam, both offered by AHIMA.

The following sections give you a brief overview of the these main certification exams. For more information on certification exams and how to prepare for them, head to Chapter 9.

## *The CPC exam (AAPC)*

To ensure that you can perform all the necessary job requirements out in the field, the CPC certification examination itself tests for strength in all areas, including the following:

- ✔ Anesthesia
- ✔ Systems of the body (head to Chapter 9 for info on those)
- ✔ Radiology
- ✔ Pathology and laboratory coding
- ✔ Medicine, including injections, psychotherapy, and other office procedures, in addition to heart catheterizations and more
- ✔ Evaluation and management service guidelines, including how to work with new patients, existing patients, consultations, and so on
- ✔ Diagnosis coding
- ✔ Medical terminology
- ✔ HCPCS codes (which relate to implants, certain *biologicals* [drugs or vaccines], and other items used in patient care)
- ✔ Coding guidelines, including bundling and modifier use (which you can read about in Chapters 11 and 12)

A reputable study program prepares you for all these areas so that you can both pass the test and perform well on the job.

To prepare for the exam, take advantage of resources offered by the AAPC. You can purchase CPC-specific study guides through the AAPC website (www.aapc.com). These study guides contain coding examples, give sample questions, and offer tips for taking the test. Practice tests designed to give you a look at actual test questions are also available to buy. The same people who made up the certification examinations prepare these simulated exams. So you're getting the inside scoop on what to expect in the testing room when you take the sample tests from the AAPC. You can also sign up for an exam review class, sponsored by local AAPC chapters (you can find these online by state and locale).

### *Prerequisites and more*

Lucky for you, you don't have to jump through a ton of prerequisite hoops before you sit down to take the CPC certification exam. In fact, the AAPC doesn't have eligibility requirements to take its certification examination, period. The organization simply advises you to be academically prepared, but you aren't required to show proof that you completed a program. Don't interpret this to mean that you should just forego your education and walk in the testing room without any prior knowledge, though. After all, you want to pass with flying colors!

The level of prior experience you have when you take the exam affects the credential you earn. To earn the full CPC designation after passing the CPC examination, you must have experience in coding. If you don't already have experience, you are eligible for only the apprentice level certification, the CPC-A. For more on what CPC-A is and how to gain full CPC designation, refer to the earlier section "The AAPC and its basic certifications: CPC, CPC-H, CPC-P."

### Test specs: Cost, format, and more

And now for the polite introductions. In this section, I cover the vital info you need to know about the test that you'll spend countless hours prepping for:

- ✔ **Cost:** You may want to start saving your pennies now. The examination cost is $300, which is hardly insignificant, especially if you're on a student budget. The good news is that, if you're enrolled in AAPC accredited programs, you qualify for a discounted fee of $260.

    Students who fail the first test are allowed one retake at no additional cost. Not that you'll need to — after all, you're going to be a coding rock star — but it's good to know you won't have to pony up another $300 if things go south.

- ✔ **Number and types of questions:** The CPC examination consists of 150 multiple-choice questions.

- ✔ **Time:** You are allowed 5 hours, 40 minutes to complete the test.

- ✔ **Resources you can use during the test:** You are allowed to use approved coding manuals as long as the writing in them (that is, your chicken scratch in the margins) doesn't contain notes such as word definitions and specialty advice from coding resources. Also, no papers can be taped or pasted inside them.

The books you can use during the test are current year and/or previous year CPT books. (Although books from the previous calendar year are allowed, the questions are based on current books, so I advise you to use current manuals instead.) You can use only the AMA standard or professional edition — not the expert edition — and no other publisher is allowed. So when it comes to CPT books in the testing room, it's AMA or the highway! You can also use officially published errata updates (which list errors in a book and furnish the appropriate revisions). As for ICD and HCPCS books, it's your call: These books don't have to be a particular edition or from a particular publisher.

The test proctors check the code books as you enter the test area. Be sure that you remove any nefarious notes before you get there. You don't want to get pinched for cheating just because you left in a note or two by accident.

- ✔ **ID:** You need a government-issued photo ID.

- ✔ **Receiving scores:** After you take the exam, the results are available online between 5 to 7 days after the proctor receives them (go to your own member area at www.aapc.com). Hardcopies of the scores are mailed within two weeks of receipt from the proctor. Unfortunately, you can't get your results by phone.

## The CCS exam (AHIMA)

The CCS examination consists of multiple-choice and fill-in-the-blank questions that are based on medical terminology and coding examples and that include questions based on pharmacology (drugs and the conditions they're prescribed to treat). You prepare for this test in the same way you prepare for the CPC examination (refer to the earlier section).

### Prerequisites and more

If you want to take the CCS examination, you must have a very basic paper in hand: your high school diploma or an equivalent like the GED. Beyond that, AHIMA recommends (but doesn't require) that you have a minimum of three years' experience in a hospital setting coding for multiple types of inpatient and outpatient cases.

AHIMA, much like the AAPC, also recommends that you are proficient in anatomy, pharmacology, and the disease processes. You'll also want to have a demonstrated proficiency in abstracting pertinent data from patient records. Why? Well, the CCS is able to assign procedure codes and the supporting diagnosis codes. Because of that, healthcare providers rely on competent coders to report data that is used for reimbursement. Also, public health agencies and research organizations use data derived from your coding patterns to identify developing needs of the industry. So your coding has lasting effects that go well beyond reimbursement for the provider.

### Test specs: Cost, format, and more

Here are the vital stats for the CCS:

- ✔ **Cost:** Currently, the cost for CCS examinations is $299 for AHIMA members and $399 for non-members — which is why it pays to be a member of AHIMA before you sign up for the CCS test. Who wants to turn down $100 savings right off the bat?

✔ **Number and types of questions:** The CCS exam consists of 81 multiple-choice questions. (Of these, 18 are considered "pre-test" questions. The pre-test questions aren't counted in your score; they're used to assess the usability of the test itself. Think of these as questions that test the test!) In addition to the multiple-choice questions, the test also includes a fill-in-the-blank portion that consists of medical record cases that you have to respond to.

✔ **Time:** The test lasts 4 hours, with no breaks. So ease up on the coffee and be sure to make time for using the restroom *before* you go in the exam room!

✔ **Resources you can use during the test:** During the test, you can use approved books (listed on the AHIMA website: www.ahima.org), but you can't use any kind of coding software, so leave that at home. Other things not allowed: cellphones or other electronic devices, food or drinks, or purses.

✔ **ID:** To get into the test, you need two forms of signed identification, at least one of which has a picture of you. Examples of acceptable IDs include a valid drivers' license, military ID, passport, Social Security card, credit or debit card, and so on. Go the AHIMA website (www.ahima.org) for more information on acceptable forms of ID.

✔ **Receiving scores:** After you take the test, you have to wait until AHIMA releases your test results, and times may vary. You can contact AHIMA directly to get an approximate turnaround time. Contact information is available on the website.

If, for some reason, you don't do as well as you'd hoped, you have to wait at least 91 days before you can apply for a re-test. The re-test requires another test fee, and you have to go through the whole application process again.

## The CCA exam (AHIMA)

As I note earlier, the CCA credential is a certification that shows you have demonstrated the ability to abstract the correct procedural and diagnosis codes in hospitals and physician practices. This credential indicates proficiency in all areas of coding, both hospital- and physician-based. Here's what you need to know:

✔ **Prerequisites:** To be eligible for this credential, you must have a high school diploma or equivalent. AHIMA also recommends that you have at least 6 months' experience working for a healthcare organization in a position that requires use of coding materials. If you don't have that experience, you must show that you've completed a formal training program instead. (An AHIMA-accredited program isn't required, but it does provide the most appropriate preparation for this examination.)

✔ **Cost:** Currently, the cost of the CCA exam is $199 for members and $299 for non-members. To find out more about the CCA, go to the AHIMA website.

# Chapter 8

# The Path to Certification: Finding a Study Program

*A*fter you familiarize yourself with the basic types of medical billing and coding certifications (the topic of the preceding chapter), you're ready to choose the right educational path to help you reach your goals. The good news about becoming a medical coder? It has fewer educational requirements than other medical careers. So you don't have to spend decades preparing for your new career. Most billing and coding programs get you up and running in a relatively short amount of time, often less than two years; having a bachelor's or master's degree is only required for some of the upper level American Health Information Management Association (AHIMA) certifications; head to Chapter 10 for more about certifications that require college degrees.

In this chapter, I explain the various educational paths open to you and highlight the things you need to know to choose the program that best suits your goals.

The certificate issued by a training program is *not* certification; it is nothing but a piece of paper saying you went through a program. True certification can only be given by one of the credentialing organizations like the AAPC (formerly known as the American Academy of Professional Coders) or AHIMA.

# The Big Picture: Thinking about Your Degree and Career Objectives

A famous proverb goes something like this: A journey of a thousand miles begins with a single step. True. But something needs to come before that first step; otherwise, you could end up going in circles or someplace you had no desire to be.

Before you begin your journey to a career as a medical biller and coder, you first need to think a bit about what you want to do.

## Prioritizing your career needs

Although you can't predict the future, you can put some thought into your long-term career needs when you're thinking about the type of training program you want. The last thing you want is to get stuck in a program that prepares you for a certification exam that doesn't match up with how you want to spend the rest of your career. As you talk your way through this decision, consider these factors:

- Where you plan to seek employment (hospital, physician's office, and so on)
- The kind of job you want to do (whether you prefer the quiet work of a coder, the data entry routine of the biller or charge poster, or the daily interaction required of account's receivable representative)
- The type of certification potential prospective employers prefer
- The availability, quality, and cost of the training programs in your area

Where you want to work and what kind of job you want to do will probably carry the most weight in your decision-making process. After all, you want to make yourself the most marketable candidate for the jobs you want most. Try these tips for tracking the ins and outs of potential employers and, by extension, the certifications they require:

- Check with local employment recruiters and see what type of credentials their clients prefer.
- Take note of the credentials displayed in local medical offices that you visit.

✔ Look through the local job listings and see what kinds of certifications are mentioned in jobs that appeal to you.

✔ If you have your heart set on working for a particular company, find out what kind of coders they prefer.

# What kind of program better meets your needs?

The type of certification(s) you want — AHIMA or AAPC, but there are others, too — may affect the type of education path you choose. Some schools cater to specific certification options, while others offer a more rounded education that focuses on the general knowledge you need to take most certification exams. So spend some time thinking about what kind of program can best prepare you for the career you want. Consider these examples:

✔ **AAPC certification** serves those individuals best who are interested in pursuing a career in physician-related coding and billing, and the AAPC certification test includes more coverage of CPT codes, the codes physician-based providers use when billing payers. (CPT stands for *current procedural terminology.*) As a result, AAPC programs cover more of the physician-specific codes than AHIMA programs do.

✔ **AHIMA credentials** are normally associated with hospital coding and billing. Its test includes more about ICD-9 Volume Three codes, which are used when billing hospital inpatient services. AHIMA programs put more emphasis on the ICD Volume Three procedure codes than AAPC programs do. (ICD stands for *International Classification of Diseases*; you can read more about ICD codes in Chapters 5 and 15.)

Don't misinterpret the distinctions between AHIMA and AAPC programs to mean that an AAPC-certified coder wouldn't be able to find work in a hospital setting or an AHIMA-certified coder couldn't work in a physician's office. Just be aware that the initial learning curve on the job may be a little steeper because the certification test is not specifically focused on the area your find yourself in.

Either program focus you choose will get you off to a solid start, so go with your gut about what best fits your goals, schedule, and learning style. If the local community college program fits your budget and schedule and happens to focus on AHIMA educational needs, then you'll likely find yourself on the AHIMA-certification path. Similarly, if the local vocational school has a well-respected AAPC-based program, you may go down the path toward AAPC certification. Either way, a job is likely waiting for you at the end of the road!

When you consider potential programs of study, keep in mind that solid medical coding and billing programs provide their students with the knowledge necessary to ace entry levels of certification. When you complete the coursework, the technical school or community college will issue you a certificate of completion. This certificate is not the same as *certification*. Although you will receive some sort of certificate or degree from your institution, you still have to take certification exams after you graduate.

## Do you want to pursue a degree?

The type of certificate or degree you earn depends entirely on the type of school you attend. Some of the community college programs offer associate's degree programs. Make sure the program you choose offers the degree you want to attain.

The degree or certificate you earn may not be as important to you as the certifications you want to master, but be mindful that getting an actual degree does have advantages:

- **It increases your earning potential.** Some employers provide better wage incentives to those with both a degree and certifications. Some employers may hire coders without any certification credentials at all, but the wage potential is greater for certified coders.

- **It increases your employment options.** The majority of billing companies are contractually obligated to employ only certified coders to perform client coding.

# Considering the Time Commitment

Time is a factor in anything you do, and it's no different when choosing a course of study. I'm going to bet that, like most people, you don't have all the time in the world to study at your leisure and take years to complete a degree. Perhaps you are embarking on a second (or third or fourth) career. Perhaps you have children or a parent to care for. Maybe you have to go to school while working at another job. Any number of time-related factors can affect what program you choose to pursue.

Looking long term, you want to consider how long you can afford to be in school — whether that means attending classes at night while you hold down a day job or taking a year off work to devote yourself 100 percent to getting your degree and certification. In the short term, you need to decide how much time you actually have available to devote to studying.

In the following sections, I walk you through some considerations to keep in mind as you create your long-term plan of action and your short-term plan of daily study.

# Planning for your time-to-degree

Although becoming certified in medical billing and coding requires only that you pass a 5-hour exam, you can expect your training to take between one and two years. Then, following certification, you should plan on an additional two years of on-the-job training. The next sections have the details.

### Time in the classroom

The amount of time you need to fully prepare for a billing and coding career depends upon your pre-existing knowledge of the field and the amount of education or training you need to prepare for a job. In general, the greater the educational or training requirements, the longer the program. If you're unfamiliar with computers or a bit rusty in your English and math skills, you may need additional classroom training to update your skill set in the basics. On the other hand, if you already work in a medial healthcare environment, you may find a program with less instruction in basic skill sets quite adequate.

Don't shortchange yourself just because you want to get through the program quickly. If one program doesn't offer training in all the skill sets you need to be successful, rule it out. Getting a little more training than you need is better than struggling because you lack the foundation necessary to process the class materials, and you'll be the better prepared candidate when the time comes to interview for jobs.

The important thing is to find a program that meets your individual needs as well as your time constraints. Don't be afraid to ask questions of school admissions counselors whose job is to find students who best fit their program. These counselors can also help you determine whether the school fits your needs in terms of time-to-degree.

### Allowing time for on-the-job training

Classroom instruction provides you with the tools of the trade, but on-the-job training teaches you how to use them. So remember to account for a year or two of this kind of training in your planning. The more experience you have in the healthcare industry prior to formal training, the shorter your post-program, on-the-job training period. For the novice with no healthcare experience, a minimum of one or two years of on-the-job training will likely be necessary.

On-the-job training is a great way to learn the nuances of billing and coding. Plus, you get paid to learn! Be sure to investigate programs that offer this as a post-grad option.

Some employers are willing to hire novice coders, but doing so can be a disservice to the novice if no onsite mentor is available. Before you say yes to a job offer straight out of school, make sure you inquire about the type of mentoring and support you can expect.

## Anticipating your day-to-day schedule

Most vocational school programs involve about 10 hours per week in the classroom. For every hour you spend in class, plan on at least 2 hours of study time. Grand total for this scenario? About 30 hours per week for class and study. But that's not all you need to consider as you think about your daily schedule. You also need to include time to commute and time for family and household responsibilities.

If you've not been in school for a while, let me offer you a refresher course in time management. Calculate approximately how many hours you need to spend on each of those activities, add them up, and then multiply that number by a factor of 10. That's how long accomplishing all these tasks each day will take. Okay, okay. I'm exaggerating. But the point is spot on: When you're in school, these tasks take longer than you anticipate. So from now on, make your mantra "Overestimate, overestimate, overestimate." Build in extra time for both study and all the other activities.

Here's some advice to help you maximize your time and stay sane in the process:

- ✔ **Dedicate ample time to study.** Regular study is essential for success. The number of hours you need depends on your current level of familiarity with the medical curriculum. If you are a registered nurse, then the only new material you'll encounter in a coding program will be the method of medical record abstraction (basically, which codes are where and how to choose them). If, on the other hand, the last time you read the word *patella* was in middle school, then mastering medical terminology and anatomy in addition to learning the methods used in coding books may require a bit more study. Plan for the scenario that's most appropriate to your situation.

- ✔ **Plan a time and place to study.** Pick a quiet time and place where you can concentrate on your work without distraction. Give your study time the same importance as your other daily tasks.

> ✔ **Take care of yourself.** Make time for ample rest and relaxation. A well-rested brain is a powerful brain. Staying up all night to study for the next day's test is counter-productive. I offer lots of study tactics in Chapter 9.

If you have a plan and the tools to study efficiently, you'll be prepared for the job, not just the test(s) and subsequent certification exams.

# Ready, Set, Prerequisites!

Nearly every course of study has a list of prerequisites, things you need to know or skill sets you need to have, to be successful as an incoming student. In the case of medical billing and coding, you don't necessarily need to know all the ins and outs of the medical industry, but you do need to sharpen your basic building-block skills — reading, keyboarding, and arithmetic, in particular — if you want to take your career to the next level. These basic requirements promote success in the classroom and on the job.

## Getting ready for your training program

General prerequisites for medical billing and coding success are strong keyboarding skills and strong reading skills. You also need to know basic math skills.

### Reading (and keyboarding) is fundamental!

To process codes clearly and effectively, you must be able to read fairly quickly, and you must have good retention. You also need to enter data accurately with a keyboard. (In billing and coding, accuracy takes preference over speed.)

Want to be a faster reader? Use a ruler to help your eyes quickly skim down a page. Want to increase your typing speed? Try one of the free online typing tutorials to refresh your fingers.

### Making the most of math

On the math side of the fence, you need to have a fairly solid proficiency in math because some positions require higher-level math skills. For example, you may have to compute reimbursements by using relative value units (RVUs) and then applying a conversion factor.

RVUs are numbers that represent the amount of work assigned to each reimbursable procedure. The conversion factor is based on the geographic location of the provider. The logic behind the conversion factor is that the overhead is higher — and it therefore costs more to run an office — in a metropolitan area (New York City, for example) than it does in a rural area (like Grover City).

To perform the math skills you'll learn in your billing and coding program, you need to have a solid grasp of math basics down first, things like addition, subtraction, and multiplication, which are part of the daily coding and billing world. Also, a basic grasp of fractions and decimals is needed for choosing the correct Healthcare Common Procedure Coding System (HCPCS) codes for specified drugs or injectables. If you're unsure about your math-related bona fides, ask your program admissions counselor about recommendations for refresher math courses at the local community college.

## Getting ready for the certification test

After you complete your training program, you're going to want to take your certification test(s). Some of these tests have prerequisites, too.

The major prerequisite for certification testing (which comes, ideally, after you complete a course of study) is a solid knowledge of medical terminology, anatomy, CPT codes and ICD-9 codes, and rules of reimbursement. As a medical biller and coder, your job is to make sure that the numbers are right when you submit them for reimbursement: the procedure code numbers, the diagnosis code numbers, the insurance policy numbers, the billing address, and every other number and letter that crosses your desk.

In addition to the preceding, other prerequisites may be necessary for AHIMA and AAPC certification. In the following sections, I explain what these prerequisites are. Before you register for these certification examinations, check out the organizations' websites — www.ahima.org and www.aapc.com — for more information about each organization's certification requirements.

### Prerequisites for AHIMA certification tests

The most basic entry-level AHIMA certifications require that you have a high school diploma or equivalent before you can sit for the examinations. Other AHIMA certification levels require bachelor's degrees or higher to sit for the certification examinations.

Medical billing and coding training programs themselves have no enrollment requirements. You can enroll, for example, fresh out of high school, after years as a stay-at-home-parent, or as a college graduate. But as I make clear in the preceding paragraph, the exams for some certification levels do have educational prerequisites. Therefore, before you enroll in a particular training program, make sure you understand the actual certification requirements that you'll encounter when you sign up for the certification tests.

### Prerequisites for AAPC certification tests

AAPC certifications don't specify high school graduation or its equivalent as a prerequisite for certification eligibility, but they do recommend it. Similarly, to take exams for specialized certification levels, the AAPC recommends that you have experience in the area of specialization prior to applying for certification.

# Picking a Program of Study

Certification may open the door to your new career, but you need to understand the workings of the industry to succeed in the billing and coding business. That's where your program of study comes in.

By attending classes and studying under professionals who know the ins and outs of the industry, you can have a competitive edge over job candidates who study independently for the certification tests.

Wherever you choose to enroll, make sure the institution offers classes in, at minimum, anatomy, medical terminology, ICD-9 coding, CPT coding, and billing practices. These subjects represent the minimum you must know to pass a certification exam and get a job in billing and coding. Ideally, full programs also offer classes that explain the different types of insurance, describe how clearinghouses operate and what their function actually is, and introduce you to the types of coding and billing software that medical practices commonly use. Your best bet is to make a list of these subject areas and keep them close by when you're looking online at potential schools or speaking with school representatives.

The path to certification can be costly; it pays to research any and all programs before making a commitment. Whether you enroll at a community college, a vocational school, or an online program, you want to weigh the pros and cons carefully to decide what best fits your needs, goals, and lifestyle so that you can move on to the next big step — taking that certification exam.

## In your backyard: Community college

Community college programs vary in cost and number of hours required for a certificate of completion.

# The ins and outs of internships and externships

Public and privately owned businesses like free or nearly free labor, and most *internships* (on-the-job training that takes place while you're in school) and *externships* (on-the-job training that takes place after you graduate) meet that definition. The businesses benefit from the work performed by the intern, and the intern benefits from the experience gained by working.

Internships are generally a result of an agreement between local businesses and local community colleges or vocational schools. The availability of these positions serves as a selling point for the school and also provides local businesses with potential employees (that's you!) who have been given the skill sets necessary to be an asset to the company.

Participating in an internship or externship has a number of benefits:

✔ **You get real on-the-job experience.** The necessary skills to become a medical coder and biller are learned in the classroom, but implementation of those skills happens on the job, and there's no substitute for job-related experience.

✔ **The exposure you receive during an internship can open the door to a paid position.** These positions often result in job offers just at a time when you're looking for a job (students serving in these positions are normally in the final steps of their respective programs or have recently completed them).

✔ **Internships and externships serve as an avenue to networking.** If you don't find employment with the current company, someone who has been working alongside you may very well know of an opening elsewhere or would be willing to serve as a professional reference in the future.

Many vocational schools have connections to the community and are able to assist with externships or internships. Check with your program's career counselors or individual instructors to find out about possible internships or externships.

*Tip:* Often instructors of the programs also work for the companies offering the internships, and the instructor's recommendation often results in the opportunity for the student. If you are interested in one of these opportunities, let your instructor (or advisor) know and then be the kind of student who gives the instructor the confidence to recommend you.

A solid community college program includes instruction in medical terminology, anatomy, physiology, and diagnosis and procedure coding. A good program also includes instruction in medical billing programs in addition to an introduction to medical clearinghouse practices.

Some community college programs send you out the door with an associate's degree, which is a diploma that usually represents completion of a two-year course of study. Others offer certificates of completion, which indicate that you have successfully completed the program. Programs offered by community colleges have both pros and cons.

### The pros of a community college

Community college billing and coding programs give you credibility because they're known to offer programs with a solid and diverse course of study. The associate's degree or certificate of completion you receive has an air of authority that you may not get from a for-profit school. Following are some other benefits:

- **Commitment to its students:** A community college is invested in the success of its alumni and often offers post-graduate services such as job search support and alumni resources for networking. Also, community college programs have ample resources to assist potential students with planning a course of study.

- **Affordability:** Community college programs are based on the normal fees of the local college; an average program costs around $2,500.00. Financial aid is usually available in the form of grants, scholarships, or loans, and the interest rate on a student loan can be quite attractive.

- **Possible externship or internship opportunity:** Many local instructors work in the industry and have the resources to offer on-the-job training opportunities.

### The cons of community college programs

Community college programs have certain drawbacks:

- **Scheduling issues:** Community college programs are usually structured to coincide with the typical college semester or session term (usually an August start for fall term and a January start date for spring). In addition, individual classes are usually structured in a series of tiers, with tier-one classes being prerequisites for the tier-two classes and so on. If life intervenes and interrupts your participation in the scheduled classes, the interruption can result in a delay of a year, which is particularly a problem when the program participation is small, because the program cycles are less frequent.

    Although you can't predict what happens in life, be sure your community college's term schedule fits with your overall lifestyle before you commit. Otherwise, you may find yourself treading water for a full year until you can take some required classes again.

- **Lack of flexibility:** As I explain in the preceding bullet, the community college curriculum is normally structured in class blocks that serve as prerequisites to the next class. The structure is such that the classes follow in order and may not offer much flexibility with regard to times and frequency. For the student already working, the lack of flexibility can be a major roadblock.

# Training the trainers

Your first priority right now is making sure you get the training that will best prepare you for the certification exam. But don't forget that the people who train you have to be trained as well.

The AAPC offers an instructor certification, Professional Medical Coding Instructor (PMCC). The individuals who hold this certification have received additional instruction above and beyond what you ultimately get, have taken a specialized teaching exam, and must have passed the certification tests they teach. These individuals are also specially licensed by the AAPC. To be eligible to take the preparation course for the exam, potential PMCCs must be members in good standing of the AAPC and have a minimum of five years of coding experience.

The preparation course itself includes instruction in understanding the process of teaching adults. The PMCC must also demonstrate a thorough knowledge of coding disciplines and their practical applications. The PMCC certification examination includes a written portion in addition to a 15-minute presentation, which is evaluated by the student's peers.

After having earned the PMCC certification, the instructor may teach accredited courses, either as an employee of a teaching institution or by offering individual instruction. So as you investigate potential training programs, be sure to sniff out who the PMCCs are in the school and make sure they're part of the staff.

✔ **Having to purchase your own books:** Many community college programs use a book rental system for students, but in a coding program, you want to keep your books so that you can use them later to study for the certification exam. Unless the cost of materials is built into your tuition, you need to purchase your own books, which can get pretty expensive. Here's why: You need the coding books to take the certification exam, and the books change every year! If the year (and coding books) changes, you need to purchase more books. The exam schedule indicates which coding books should be used to find the right answers.

*Note:* Procedure codes that are found in the CPT book are added and deleted annually, and the ICD-9 books add new diagnosis codes every year. In addition, in October 2014, the United States will transition from ICD-9 to ICD-10. This major change will affect every diagnosis code that billers and coders use. Guess what that means — you'll need to buy more books!

If you use an older book (say, one you buy from an online reseller) while you're in school or to take your certification exam, it may not do much damage. But in the actual work of coding, numbers are everything. After you begin your job, you absolutely must use the right book.

# *Vocation station: Technical school programs*

Vocational schools offer an alternative to the community college route. Some of these programs offer excellent training. In the following sections, I go over some of the most common pros and cons of technical school programs.

### *The pros of a technical school*

Attending a vocational or technical school program offers certain advantages:

- ✔ **The programs are usually more subject specific and take less time to complete.** The more specialized vocational programs usually focus on subject matter that is directly related to the program, such as medical terminology, anatomy, how to use coding materials, understanding insurance, and an introduction of various coding and billing software programs. They also tend to cycle more often (that is, the programs are offered more frequently), which eliminates a longer waiting time to begin a program.

  Although the abbreviated course schedule means less time from enrollment to certificate of completion, don't assume that it means less commitment to study. If the program is complete but shorter, you have less time to learn the material because you're covering the same amount in a shorter timeframe, which may translate to a greater need for out-of-class study time.

- ✔ **The specialized curriculum makes for smaller classes and promotes more interaction with the instructors.** This is a bonus for you as a student. More face time equals more personal instruction.

- ✔ **Vocational and technical schools often have lower out-of-pocket costs.** Many vocational programs include coding materials with the cost of tuition, and many of the AAPC programs also include a student membership and the certification examination fee. This represents a significant out-of-pocket savings (the cost of a typical certification exam is $300 — $260 for students with student memberships — and the books at a bundled price are about $160). A student membership is offered at a discount to individuals enrolled in an AAPC-accredited program. Yes, you're still paying for these items through tuition payments, but it tends to hurts less when it's all rolled into one payment.

  *Note:* Having lower out-of-pocket expenses doesn't necessarily mean that these programs are less expensive. In fact, they may be more expensive. The next section has the details.

### *The cons of technical schools*

Following are the disadvantages of vocational or technical school programs:

- ✔ **Vocational school programs often are more costly.** Unlike community colleges, vocational schools are purely self-supporting and for-profit institutions. Programs may cost closer to $10,000 (this cost usually includes material costs and the fees to sit for a certification examination).

  Make sure exam fees are included in your tuition and that, at the end of the program, you can take the certification exam as an inclusive part of your paid program. (A major marketing tactic these programs use is to boast that 90 percent of their graduates receive certification upon completion, which is one reason the cost of the exam is rolled into the tuition. The thinking is that students are more likely to study for and take an exam that they've already paid for.)

- ✔ **You likely have to fly solo when seeking financial aid.** As for-profit institutions, technical schools aren't structured like a typical college or community college, meaning they often have no financial aid office to support students. If you need financial aid, you need to seek grants, scholarships, and loans on your own.

- ✔ **They may not be accredited.** Unfortunately, as the field of medical coding and billing rapidly grows, so do the number of scams and diploma mills. The onus is on you to seek out accredited programs that require study in the necessary topics. To find out how to tell good programs from bad, head to the later section "Caveat Emptor: Watching Out for Diploma Mills."

## *Clicking the mouse: Online training*

You can prepare for a career in medical coding and billing through an online program. If you're self-motivated or if you're already working in the medical field, online training may be just what you need. Like the community college and vocational school programs, online study has advantages and disadvantages, which I explain in the following sections.

Online education is no substitute for student-instructor interaction, but it is a good alternative for people who already have a billing and coding knowledge base and want to go it alone.

## A bundle of joy, courtesy of AAPC

The AAPC offers an Online Bundle for both CPC or CPC-H courses of study (see Chapter 7 for specifics on these certifications). The bundle includes the following:

✔ An online preparation course that teaches necessary coding skills for the specified area (CPC or CPC-H) and prepares the student for the certification examination. The course is designed to be completed in four months or less.

✔ Course-related materials, including a textbook and accompanying workbook. **Note:** These are not coding books; you must purchase those separately.

✔ Up to three practice examinations.

✔ The cost of taking the certification examination. You must take it within one year of enrolling in the course.

You can find out more about this bundle training at www.aapc.com.

AHIMA also offers an online training program, called the Coding Basics Program. This 12-course program is broken down into clusters that are made up of specific courses. The program is more in-depth than other online programs and is structured closely to instructor-led classrooms. To enroll in the online program, you must meet the prerequisite: proof of a C grade or better in a college-level, basic human anatomy and physiology course, or completion of AHIMA's qualifying course. You can find more information about the program on the AHIMA website at www.ahima.org.

Although a novice is eligible to enroll in either of these programs, the programs are really a better choice for individuals who are already familiar with healthcare.

### Pros of online programs

Here are the advantages that an online program has to offer:

✔ **Scheduling flexibility:** The biggest advantage online study provides is flexibility. With online studies, you attend classes at your own convenience. A quality online study program sets deadlines for completing the classwork, but it's up to you to work it around your schedule. You decide when to log in for class, be it noon or midnight. You just log in and go, which is a great benefit if you have a full-time job, kids, or other responsibilities that don't allow you to participate in a typical day-to-day class schedule.

✔ **Access to programs regardless of your location:** Online programs are not geographically restrictive. You don't have to live in an urban area to enroll in a training program. You can live on the North Pole and attend class via an online portal. Having access to any online program is especially beneficial if you live in a rural area or don't have reliable transportation to a college campus.

✔ **Less costly:** Online programs tend to be less costly than community college or vocational programs due, in part, to the fact that the school has less overhead. Fewer needs for physical facilities, resources, and higher faculty salaries help lower the costs for online programs. Plus, many online programs are a cog in the wheel of a larger bricks-and-mortar institution, so on-campus or commuter student tuition already covers much of the overhead, allowing for lower costs for online participants.

### Cons of online programs

Although saving big bucks and going to class in your jammies are real boons, online programs have some obvious drawbacks:

✔ **You have limited access to educational support:** Online students must be able to work independently and without the structure provided by a traditional classroom. With online instruction, you have less student-teacher interaction. If you're working at 3 a.m. and have a question, for example, an instructor is probably not going to be available for a discussion. Although you may be able to communicate with your instructor via message boards or e-mail, you'll still need to wait for an answer before you can proceed with your assignment.

Mastering the art of self-directed learning can be a challenge for some. It can be especially frustrating for a student who is unfamiliar with the healthcare industry. Online instruction is probably a better choice for a student who is already working in healthcare. Access to a mentor is an asset that isn't always included with online tuition.

✔ **You need to be technically savvy.** Online students need to be able to correct the myriad issues that arise when working online. Let's face it: How many times do you forget to hit "Save?" To succeed online, you need to know your hardware, your software, and the quirks that go along with them. If locating the Power button is the extent of your technical knowledge, you may want to steer clear of the online option.

✔ **Online programs have a higher incidence of being scam operations.** Do not enroll in an online program that is not accredited by either the AAPC or AHIMA. The same organizations that lend credibility to vocational programs also have tools that allow you to verify the credibility of online programs, and the same organization accreditation standards apply to online programs as classroom training.

Quality online programs offer the same curriculum as any accredited programs. They also allow students to communicate directly with the instructor, either through live chat sessions or e-mail. Although the communication isn't face-to-face, the level of accessibility with your instructor should be the same as it would be in a typical classroom setting. For more things to look at when investigating the credibility of a program, head to the later section "Caveat Emptor: Watching Out for Diploma Mills."

✔ **You have less opportunity to network with other students and faculty.** Don't care about the social aspect? Think about this: Who would you be more likely to recommend: your online classmate or the person sitting in the next desk?

If you enroll in an online program, locate the local professional chapter of the credentialing organization you want to join and start attending the meetings. Doing so is a great way to add the networking component that online programs lack. You can locate local chapters through the national organization websites or by calling the AAPC (800-626-CODE [2633]) or AHIMA (312-233-1100).

✔ **Materials necessary to complete program can be costly.** Online programs usually require that you purchase coding books just like community college programs do, so the costs can add up. Unfortunately, you can't get coding books in many places, and the only discounts you can get are by purchasing bundles; see the sidebar "A bundle of joy, courtesy of AAPC," earlier in this chapter for details.

✔ **Certification exam costs are not included in the program cost.** Certification exams can be costly (refer to Chapter 7), and as I explain earlier, you need the most current materials when you take the tests. Unlike programs offered at vocational schools, the cost of the exam probably won't be included with your online tuition. So be prepared to pony up the costs after you get through your online program.

# Caveat Emptor: Watching Out for Diploma Mills

One of the biggest drawbacks to the increasing need for billers and coders is the rise of programs that are nothing but diploma mills. These unscrupulous companies take your money and leave you with a piece of paper but no true marketability. Here are some clues that the program isn't a good one:

✔ Their ads claim that, in just a few weeks time, you'll be operating your own business out of your home, and clients will be beating down your door. Reputable medical billing and coding programs may tout some of the ways you can use a degree, but they don't make big promises about riches and fame.

✔ They promise that you can get certification of completion with a minimal amount of study or classwork. Quality programs — whether college, vocational, or online — require both classroom time and self-study time. In addition, the material covered is similar across the board and includes instruction in anatomy, medical terminology, coding, insurance rules for both Medicare and commercial insurers, and billing software programs.

How do you tell a credible program from ones that are just scams? Start by checking with AHIMA and the AAPC. Both organizations' websites list accredited training programs, those that offer the correct curriculum, have instructors certified to teach, and use a curriculum that follows the guidelines established by the organization. For more on each organization's accreditation criteria, go to their websites: AHIMA (www.ahima.org) and AAPC (www.aapc.com). Both organizations also have search tools that assist in finding certified training programs. These groups can recommend a program that fits your needs without taking you to the bank.

If your researching schools on your own, get answers to these questions:

- How long has the school been in business?
- Is the school accredited?
- How many students are in each class, and what is the student-to-teacher ratio?
- Can you reach the instructor outside of class?
- If the curriculum does not suit you, what is the refund policy?
- Does the school have a placement department to help graduates find jobs?
- What is the program's placement rate for graduates?
- What are the credentials of the instructors, and what is the ratio of full time versus adjunct instructors?

You can also ask to see the school's business license. In addition, legitimate schools have financial aid advisors to assist prospective students with finding a way to finance their training. Ideally, the financial aid pays for books and supplies. Some grants even pay for room and board. These financial aid packages are the same ones that community college and four-year-college students are given.

If the school representative seems less than truthful or tries to convince you that, after six weeks, students are suddenly inundated with job offers, walk away. If the representative tells you that completion of the program prepares students to open a home office and start a business, *run* away. These are all signs of diploma mills. Another indication that the school is a possible scam is that it has changed its name several times or has moved from state to state.

Bottom line: If it smells fishy or sounds too good to be true, it is.

# Chapter 9

# Signing Up and Preparing for the Certification Exam

. . . . . . . . . . . . . . . . . . . . . . . . . . . . . . . . . . . . . . . . . . . . .

*In This Chapter*

▶ Setting up a study routine

▶ Sharpening your focus on specific topics

▶ Reviewing ways to relieve pre-test jitters

▶ Registering for the exam

. . . . . . . . . . . . . . . . . . . . . . . . . . . . . . . . . . . . . . . . . . . . .

The time to rock that certification exam is near! You've taken the classes (if you haven't, Chapter 8 helps you find a study program), and you've determined the type of exam you want to take (see Chapter 7 for a breakdown of different tests). Now, the only thing left for you to do is study, study, and study some more before you sign up for that exam and ace it.

In this chapter, I provide all sorts of advice to help you make the most of your study time and stay sane while you do it. I also tell you what you need to know to sign up for the exam(s).

## Establishing a Study Routine and Strategy

The saying "Work smarter, not harder" truly applies to certification exam study techniques. To do well, you need to comprehend a lot of material, so much so, in fact, that you'll be better off if you prioritize what you need to study and when. Your success in a medical and billing program depends on your ability to learn new material quickly and efficiently.

Everyone had his or her individual style of studying, but certain techniques have proven to be effective. One of the best ways to increase retention, for example, is to do the assigned reading, listen as the material is discussed, and then make notes that translate the material into your own words.

Understanding what kind of learner you are is helpful, too. Are you a visual learner, someone who remembers what she sees? Or are you an auditory learner, remembering what you hear? Maybe you learn best when you can associate movement with concepts. Whatever your learning style, practice retention exercises in a way that best suits you. Whether you use flashcards, podcasts, videos, or write out your own study notes, go with what works for you.

Before you dig into those books, though, you've got to carve out some space, both physically and mentally, and you have to make time, which I discuss in the next sections. After all, your success is directly related to the advance planning you do and the amount of work and energy you invest in your studies.

## Setting up your own space

Efficient study requires concentration, so you need to set aside a space to do just that, even if all you can find in your house is a quiet corner of the living room. Here are some pointers:

- **Choose an area that works for you.** If you're like many people who believe that they study better and retain more if they simulate a class-room environment, choose an area that lets you sit at a desk or table in a firm chair. If you're more likely to curl up in a chair to study, make sure the chair isn't so comfortable that you fall asleep.

- **Select an area that's free of distractions.** When you're preparing to take a test, you want all your senses directed toward the thinking process.

    Some people find background music helpful when they study, but that doesn't mean playing music that makes you want to sing along. As soon as you start to sing along — or even become aware of the music — you're distracted and not putting all your attention on your studies.

- **Set up the study area with the necessary supplies.** You should have paper, pencils, highlighters, ruler, and a trash can nearby so that you don't have to go hunting for these things when you need them.

- **As often as time allows, study in your designated study area.** By using a familiar environment to study and then test, you can recall material more easily.

## Clearing your calendar for study

As you progress through the program on your way to the big exam, keep track of important dates. Most course schedules indicate the dates on which topics are to be introduced and when the big certification test is scheduled. With this info, you can rearrange your schedule to avoid conflicts with other activities and set aside the time necessary to study.

Last-minute cram sessions make life stressful and don't help you learn the material. In addition, memorizing material just to pass a test isn't in your best interest. To bill and code correctly on the job, you need to know all the material they teach you. It's not like you can forget anatomy or diagnosis codes when the test is over. Every course taught in a coding program and everything covered in the certification test are essential to the revenue cycle process.

To be a successful biller and coder, you must understand the body, the disease process, and illness and injury, all of which require a foundation in human anatomy and physiology. Without this foundational knowledge, the medical terminology is nothing more than random words. You may be able to link key words to the correct procedural and diagnosis codes, but when you have to fully decipher an operative report and abstract all reportable procedures, you'll be in trouble. So in your long-term test prep planning and calendar clearing, allow ample time for the proper instruction.

## Developing a study strategy

When you finally score some dedicated space in your house and time on your calendar, you can sit down and start studying. But, you say, "Where do I start? There is *so much* information!" True, you do need to know a lot (I give you a brief overview of the key topics in the next section, "Focusing on the Right Topics"). Here, I list some helpful study techniques and strategies that can help you retain important information:

- ✔ **Focus on the key ideas and concepts.** How do you know what these are? Simply look over the review exercises at the end of a chapter or section before you begin reading. By looking at the review questions first, you'll be more focused on the main ideas of the assignment as you read.

  **Use a ruler as you read.** Doing so helps you read faster and stay focused. Plus, much of the material you're studying may be completely foreign to you, which means you can easily skip lines without being aware that you're doing so.

- ✔ **Rewrite the key ideas in your own words.** If you understand the topic enough that you can explain it in your own words, you're good to go.

- ✔ **Mark up your books.** When you come to something important in the text, use a highlighter to make it stand out. Write notes in the margins to serve as reminders.

  Anatomy books are full of diagrams and illustrations. Pay special attention to how these relate to the text and make any notes that can help you remember.

Although you can and should make notes in your coding books, keep in mind that books you use on your certification examinations can't have definitions or notes that supplement other parts of the examination. For example, when you're taking the medical terminology portion of the exam, your notes in the CPT or ICD books shouldn't have terminology definitions.

✔ **Regularly review topics you studied previously.** If you don't have much time to devote to studying on a particular day, use what time you do have for review of past lessons. If you mark up your textbook as I suggest in the preceding bullet item, you don't need to re-read the old chapters entirely; you can hit the highlights, literally!

## You say "tomato" ... Learning proper pronunciation

It's no secret that many of the words you encounter in the billing and coding world don't exactly roll off the tongue (consider *acetabulum* or *olecranon!*), and mispronouncing these terms can be an embarrassment. Worse, people — like hiring managers — may take your mispronunciations to mean that you don't know the subject matter. Learning the correct pronunciation of medical terminology gives you credibility.

Although a knowledgeable instructor can educate you about correct pronunciation, another alternative is the interactive CD that some textbook publishers provide with their printed materials. These discs are a great way to learn correct pronunciation of medical terminology because you can work with it at your leisure.

Some interactive CDs phonetically pronounce the word parts (prefixes and suffixes; see Chapter 5) and then put the word together; these are wonderful learning tools.

Several solid anatomy and physiology resources are available for billing and coding students, many of which offer online access or interactive CDs. Here are my top three:

✔ *Gray's Anatomy for Students: With STUDENT CONSULT Online Access,* **by Richard L. Drake, A. Wayne Vogl, and Adam W.M. Mitchell:** This book sets the standard for medical reference materials. It includes illustrations that are a huge asset to any classroom anatomy lesson. Purchasing the book gives you access to the online version of the book, which includes interactive exercises.

✔ *Anatomy and Physiology Revealed Version 2.0 CD,* **by the University of Toledo:** An interactive CD that uses cadaver photos, this resource lets you study the body by peeling away layers to view underlying structures. It also has audio pronunciations and quizzes.

✔ *Atlas of Human Anatomy: With Student Consult Access,* by Frank H. Netter, MD. This book uses detailed illustrations to assist you with both vocabulary and anatomy. It also includes an online access pin number, which offers additional learning resources.

# Focusing on the Right Topics

To learn everything you need to know in the time you have available, you need to focus your study. Otherwise, you'll be the academic equivalent of a chicken with its head cut off, just running around all crazy-like.

The good news is that the certification test you take pretty much determines the information you need to know. Beyond that, all certification examinations assess competency in all areas of health information. You can be sure that your training program (see Chapter 8) is going to prepare you for questions covering many the primary billing and coding subject areas, such as

✔ Medical terminology

✔ Human body systems, their structure, and normal function

✔ Disease process and various treatments

## Identifying body systems

The majority of medical billing and coding training programs begin with basic human anatomy and physiology, more commonly referred to as *body systems.* You need to understand how each organ within a particular body system works, how disease or illness affects the system, and why the treatment was necessary.

Most textbooks contain diagrams specific to each body system. These diagrams show the organs within each system and describe the function of each organ as it relates to the individual system. In addition, you'll see illustrations showing cells, tissues, and several different types of disease processes. As you read the text, closely study the illustrations. Doing so not only clarifies the general concepts, but it also reinforces the information. The human body has 10 systems, each of which is made up of specialized organs that must work together for the human body to function properly and efficiently. When one system is affected by illness, all the other systems are affected in some way. I give you a quick introduction to the systems of the human body in the following sections.

A solid foundation in human anatomy and physiology is a huge asset when taking the certification examination. In fact, it's a prerequisite for most American Health Information Management Association (AHIMA)–accredited programs and is suggested (but not required) for AAPC (formerly, the American Academy of Professional Coders) programs. But knowing human anatomy and physiology is important for more than just passing the test. Without a thorough understanding in anatomy, you'll have a difficult time locating the correct procedural codes. After all, you need to know which part of the body is being treated so you can apply the proper codes.

### The circulatory system

The circulatory system transports nutrients and gasses to all cells of the body. There are two parts of this system:

- ✔ **The cardiovascular system** is composed of the heart, blood vessels, and blood (see Figure 9-1).

- ✔ **The lymphatic system** is made up of the lymph nodes, *lymphatic vessels* (which carry the lymph fluid), the *thymus* (the gland that helps produce T-cells, which are a type of white blood cell), and the spleen, as well as other parts (see Figure 9-2).

### The digestive system

The digestive system, shown in Figure 9-3, converts food into nutrients that the body can use (or *metabolize*). The primary organs of this system are the mouth, stomach, intestines (small and large), and the rectum. The system's accessory organs (organs that assist the system in performing its function) are the teeth, tongue, liver, and pancreas.

### The endocrine system

The endocrine system maintains growth and *homeostasis* (a fancy way of saying the body's "status quo"). It is made up of the pituitary gland, *pineal gland* (the gland that secretes melatonin, the hormone that regulates the sleep-wake cycle), thyroid gland, hypothalamus, adrenal glands, and ovaries in the female and testes in the male, as well as some other parts. Figure 9-4 shows the endocrine system.

### The integumentary system

The integumentary system protects the internal organs from damage, protects the body from dehydration, and stores fat. It is made of skin, hair, nails, and sweat glands.

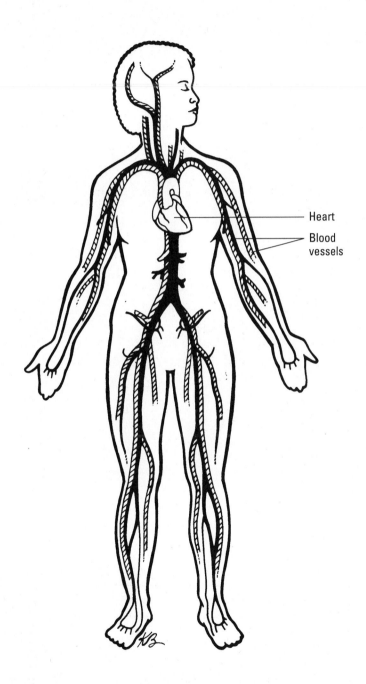

Heart

Blood
vessels

**Figure 9-1:**
The cardio-
vascular
system, the
heart of the
circulatory
system.

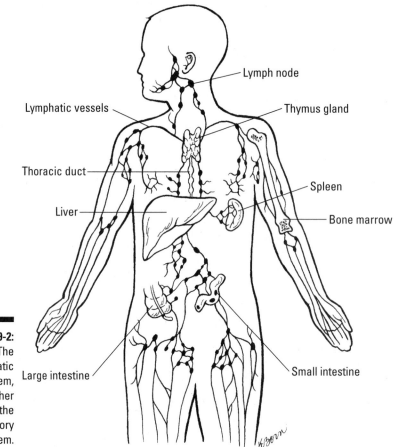

**Figure 9-2:**
The
lymphatic
system,
another
part of the
circulatory
system.

Lymph node

Lymphatic vessels

Thymus gland

Thoracic duct

Liver

Spleen

Bone marrow

Large intestine

Small intestine

### *The musculoskeletal system*

The musculoskeletal system is made up of two systems: the skeletal system and the muscular system.

The skeletal system protects the body and gives it its shape and form. It's made up of bones, joints, *ligaments* (fibers that connect bones to other bones), *tendons* (fibers that connect muscles to bones), and cartilage. The muscular system is made up of — you guessed it — muscles, tendons, ligaments, and cartilage. It enables the body to move. The muscular system has three kinds of muscles:

- ✔ **Cardiac muscle:** This is the heart muscle.

- ✔ **Smooth, or *involuntary*, muscles:** These muscles make up several internal organs. They're called involuntary muscles because we don't control their movements (the movement of the intestinal walls, for example).

- ✔ **Skeletal, or *voluntary*, muscles:** These muscles allow us to move. They're called voluntary muscles because we control them.

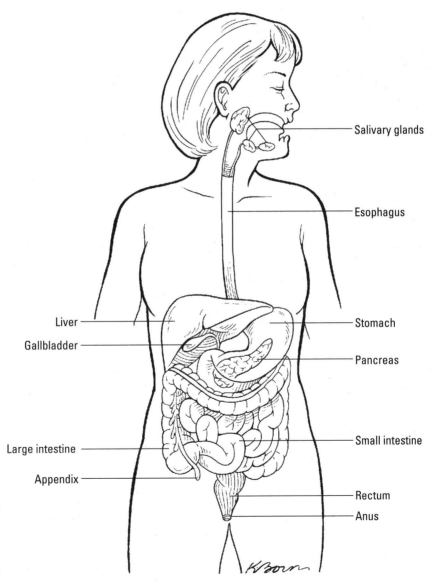

**Figure 9-3:**
The digestive system.

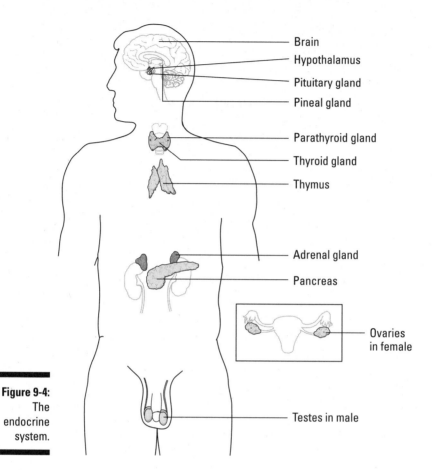

Brain
Hypothalamus
Pituitary gland
Pineal gland

Parathyroid gland
Thyroid gland
Thymus

Adrenal gland
Pancreas

Ovaries
in female

Testes in male

**Figure 9-4:**
The
endocrine
system.

### The nervous system

The nervous system monitors the internal (body temperature, pulse rate, and so on) and external (sights, sounds, and smells) environment and sends messages to the individual organs or systems to respond accordingly. It is made of the brain, spinal cord, and nerves. Messages travel from the brain down the spinal cord to nerve receptors throughout the body.

### The reproductive system

The reproductive system enables the production of offspring. The male reproductive system is made up of the testes, scrotum, penis, *vas deferens* (the passage way for sperm), and prostate. The female reproductive system is made up of the ovaries, fallopian tubes, uterus, and vagina. The mammary glands are considered accessory organs.

### The respiratory system

The respiratory system provides oxygen to all cells of the body by performing gas exchanges between air and blood gases. It is made up of the nose, trachea, lungs, and *bronchi* (the main passages of the trachea that leads to the lungs), as well as other parts (see Figure 9-5).

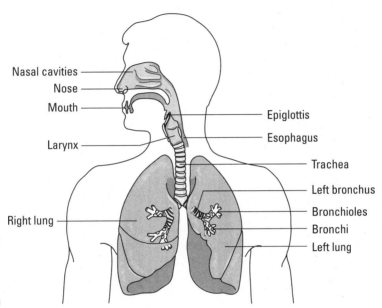

Nasal cavities

Nose

Mouth

Epiglottis

Esophagus

Larynx

Trachea

Left bronchus

Bronchioles

Right lung

Bronchi

Left lung

**Figure 9-5:**
The respiratory system.

### The urinary/excretory system

The urinary/excretory system, shown in Figure 9-6, removes wastes and maintains water balance in the body. It is made up of the kidneys, urinary bladder, *urethra* (the passage from the bladder that transports urine outside of the body), and *ureters* (the passages from the kidneys to the bladder).

## Understanding medical terminology

The coding certification examination is an assessment of your readiness to be a medical coder. All the components of the certification program are targeted toward this exam. Your knowledge of medical terminology is part of the assessment, as well as an integral part of understanding all the other things you need to know, both to pass the exam and to succeed on the job. Remember, the AAPC exam contains a specific section on medical terminology. The AHIMA exams are a little different, but they still require a solid understanding of the terminology used in the healthcare profession.

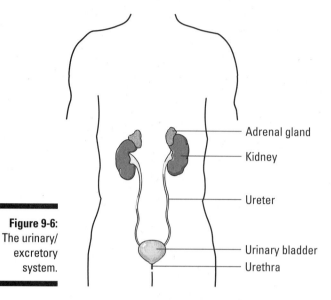

**Figure 9-6:**
The urinary/
excretory
system.

Adrenal gland

Kidney

Ureter

Urinary bladder

Urethra

Why is a firm knowledge of medical terminology so important? Why not just look up the words you need? Because doing so will take you about five times as long to do your job. Before you can assign an ICD-9 diagnosis code to an illness or injury, you need to be able to identify it in the medical record. Physicians are trained to provide diagnosis verbiage in all patient records. Your job is to abstract the correct diagnosis and procedural codes by translating the verbiage in the medical record. Knowing the prefixes and suffixes and how they work together will clue you in to what you need to know to properly code a procedure.

When you study the terminology, pay attention to the prefixes and suffixes, most of which are Greek or Latin in origin. Here's a quick heads-up on what you need to pay attention to (see Chapter 5 for more details on how to decipher medical terms):

✔ **Prefixes:** The prefix, or beginning part of a word, gets you started with understanding what is going on. It normally tells you where in the body something was done. If the first part of the word, for example, is *nephro-*, which means "kidney," you know that the relevant body part is the kidney.

When billing and coding, you want the diagnosis prefixes and the procedural prefixes to match up. For example, if the record were to contain the word *tarsal* and then switch to *carpal*, you'd want to investigate, because *carpal* means "hand" and *tarsal* means "foot." Big, big difference.

✔ **Suffixes:** The suffix, the ending part of a term, usually indicates what was done or how it was done. There are fewer suffixes than prefixes, but they are essential when identifying the correct codes to be submitted for reimbursement. For example, *-ectomy* (surgical removal), *-otomy* (surgical opening), and *-ostomy* (opening) are all similar, but they have entirely different meanings.

 A good way to learn prefixes and suffixes is to use index cards. With this method, you can assemble words, mix and match, and form a solid under-standing of the meaning of each word part and, eventually, the complete term.

## Boning up on insurer and payer rules

Although a small part of coding certification, knowing the insurer and payer rules is a big part of biller certification. In that arena, you want to be familiar with the basic filing requirements and the different types of claim forms for commercial and government payers. You also need to know when modifi-ers are necessary (and when they're not) and how to use them. For general information on when and how to use modifiers correctly, head to Chapter 12. Payer-specific filing requirements are usually found in the contract or may be found in the payer's policies (located on the payer's website).

# On Approach: Getting Ready for the Big Day

Even if you know what topics to expect on the exam, have adopted all my study suggestions, and have practiced, gone over, and reviewed all your notes and books, a couple things may still trip you up when the time comes to actually take your certification exams. Those things? Stress (your mind doesn't work so well when it's frozen in panic) and improper notes in your coding books (which means you can't use the book you've been counting on during your exam). In the next sections, I tell you how to avoid either scenario.

## Finding ways to stress less

If you are one of those people who suffers from test anxiety, in the follow-ing sections, I share some test-taking strategies that may help you feel less stress.

### Doing one, last review of coursework

If you take the advice I give earlier in this chapter and budget your time so that you have sufficient time to study, you're already ahead of the game. When exam time approaches, do the following:

✔ Ask your instructor to specify the areas that will be emphasized on the test. Focus on these areas during your final review.

✔ Review any material from practice tests, workbook exercises, sample coding exercises, review material, the textbook, and class notes.

✔ Make sure you're familiar with the way the sections are arranged in your ICD-9 and CPT books.

The materials you've been using to practice your coding skills, the ICD-9 and CPT books, are the same materials you use for the certification examination. So make sure you're familiar with how and where to look for the information that you need. You can find more on this topic in the section "Knowing how to use your resources."

✔ Review your practice tests results and make sure you understand any errors you made. Remember: Each test you take helps prepare for the next. For more on where to get practice tests, head to the section "Signing Up for and Taking the Big Test."

### Tricks to avoid — or reduce — stress

Here are a few things you can do to stay as stress-free as possible:

✔ Make a list of materials you need — everything from pencils and code books — and get these things ready the night before so that you don't have to rush around searching for them the day of the exam.

✔ Wear comfortable clothing and arrive early for the examination.

✔ Keep a positive mindset that you're going to do your best.

✔ Don't pay too much attention to the other test-takers. Stress can be contagious.

## Knowing how to use your resources

As the test time nears, look through your ICD-9 and CPT books. Make sure you're familiar with all the sections and highlight the areas you want to focus on. If you prefer, you can put identifying tabs on the book to help remember different sections. (**Note:** Professionals don't tab their books. Books with tabs imply a lack of experience and familiarity with the material. Tabs are fine for the test, but remove them after you clear that hurdle.)

Here's how to use these resources effectively:

1. **First look in the ICD-9 index to find the diagnosis; then go to that section of the book, called the *tabular list*, to identify the corresponding diagnosis code.**

Make sure that you don't leave off a fourth or fifth digit. The ICD-9 book guides you to the correct diagnosis code but may not provide the complete diagnosis code. So don't try to save time and code from the index. Always code from the tabular list.

2. **After you have the diagnosis code, refer to the CPT book for the procedural code(s).**

   Determine which part of the body the procedure(s) involved; then refer to that section of the CPT book.

   The CPT book has an index, but it's not particularly useful when you're looking for procedures. For that reason, look directly in the appropriate section of the book to identify the code that reflects the procedures.

3. **Check to make sure that the diagnosis code supports medical necessity for the procedural code you're submitting.**

   For example, if you are reporting a hernia repair, make sure that the diagnosis is a hernia.

The test proctors examine all materials brought into the testing area. Make sure you haven't written any notes in your CPT and ICD-9 book that will bar you from using them during the exam. Highlighted areas are acceptable, and personal notes may be okay, but definitions of medical terms aren't. If you've noted something like "measles, mumps, rubella" next to MMR vaccine, you either need to erase it or use a book the proctor provides. Also forbidden are notes that involve information from sources other than the approved coding materials. (This is another reason to attend local chapter meetings. The examination proctors are normally chapter officers, and they're more than happy to advise you with regard to the acceptability of your books.)

Here are some other things not allowed into the test areas: reference or study materials, post-it notes, loose-leaf paper notes, calculators, cell phones, or any materials that give you an unfair advantage.

# Signing Up for and Taking the Big Test

When you decide that the time is right to take the certification examination, check the website of the organization whose test you have prepared to take. AHIMA has testing information on its website (www.ahima.org), and AAPC has the necessary information on its website (www.aapc.com).

The training program you enroll in will direct you to its certification examinations. If your program does not include certification testing arrangements, you need to register and pay for any and all examinations that you plan to take.

Plan ahead! Both AHIMA and AAPC require prepaid registration several weeks in advance of the scheduled examinations. In addition, the tests are scheduled at the convenience of the certification organizations. Although they are available year-round, a limited number of seats are available at each session. The tests are also dependent upon volunteer proctors whose time is to be respected. Oh, and don't be late! Proctors lock the door before the test begins, and no one is allowed in after that point.

Both organizations offer practice tests that you can purchase prior to the actual examination. Consider taking one to see how you do. In addition, local AAPC chapters often hold review classes before an exam to help those taking the exam practice their skill and timing. Experienced officers or other members with a solid background in teaching often lead these classes.

In the following sections, I give you a general idea of the kinds of questions you can expect, explain when you can expect your score, and offer several test-taking tips.

## *Taking a quick peek at the exam*

The tests are shipped to the exam proctor prior to the testing date. The seal on each test remains unbroken until the examinee is ready to begin or you're given permission to begin. Then you're allowed a specified amount of time to complete the exam (5 hours and 40 minutes for AAPC's CPC test, for example, and 4 hours for AHIMA's CCS exam). The test format is multiple-choice or a combination of multiple-choice and fill-in-the-blank.

Following are some examples of possible types of questions that may be on the certification examination(s).

A section on medical terminology will ask questions such as

> What does MMR stand for?
>
> What is the meaning of homeostasis?
>
> What is a ROS?
>
> What is an H&P?
>
> What is medical necessity?

The section on human anatomy may include questions such as

> What are the parts of the circulatory system?
>
> Are the bronchi part of the (A) skeletal system, (B) muscle system, (C) integumentary system, or (D) respiratory system?

The spleen is an organ found in the _____system.

The Achilles tendon is part of the _____.

The metacarpal is found in which part of the body?

Also expect to find coding-specific questions that ask you to identify the correct diagnosis code(s) as indicated by the terminology in the question. Here are some examples:

What is the correct ICD-9 code for carpal tunnel syndrome: (A) 354.0, (B) 354.2, (C) 354.3, or (D) none of the above?

What is the correct ICD-9 code for closed fracture radius alone unspecified part: (A) 813.00, (B) 813.30, (C) 813.24, or (D) none of the above?

Does ICD-9 diagnosis code 733.82 represent (A) mal-union or (B) non-union?

In which section of the CPT book is a splenectomy found?

An arthroscopic left knee medial meniscectomy is CPT _____.

Chondroplasty is always included with arthroscopic knee procedures. True or False?

You may also be presented with scenarios that ask you to employ your coding skills. Here's an example scenario:

Pre-operative diagnosis: left Achilles tendon rupture. Post-operative diagnosis: Same. Procedure: Left Achilles tendon repair.

Consent was obtained and the patient received a regional block prior to administration of general anesthesia. A tourniquet was placed on the left thigh and inflated. An 8 cm longitudinal incision was made over the rupture. Sharp dissection was used to tunnel through the subcutaneous tissue to expose the rupture. Two #2 fiber wires were used to repair the tendon. The incision was then closed with 0-vicryl, the tourniquet was deflated, and the dermis was closed in the usual fashion.

Please supply diagnosis and procedure codes for the above.

For specific information about the kinds of questions you'll find on either the AAPC exams or the AHIMA exams, refer to Chapter 7.

## Making the grade — or not

A passing score for the exams is 70 percent or above. Test scores are usually available in six to eight weeks and are sent by mail, or you can ask to receive them via e-mail.

If you don't do well on the certification exam despite all your prep, you can re-take the test. The AAPC allows one re-take without additional fees, although you do have to register for the examination again, just as for the initial sitting. If you need to take the AHIMA test again, you must pay the fee again, as well.

## Test-taking tips

Successful test-taking requires careful preparation and the ability to avoid making careless mistakes. Following are some tips that can help you ensure that you get the highest score possible:

- ✔ **Carefully read the directions for each section.** Doing so helps you avoid careless errors.

- ✔ **Quickly look through each section of the test for an overview and scan for keywords.** The keyword identifies which part of the body is being treated.

- ✔ **Answer the easy questions first to build confidence; then go back and answer more difficult ones.** If you get stuck on an answer, skip it and come back to it later if time permits. Don't stress over one question and ignore others you may know.

- ✔ **On the multiple-choice questions, eliminate obvious incorrect answers.** Then choose the best option from those remaining.

- ✔ **On the operative note section, read carefully and note the primary procedure first.** Then note the diagnosis that supports medical necessity.

- ✔ **Don't leave blanks.** A non-answer is an incorrect answer, so if you are not sure, guess.

- ✔ **If you have extra time, check your answers.** Resist the urge to leave immediately after you complete the test. Check to make sure that you have answered all the questions and that you haven't mismarked any answers.

As you go along, you may come across information in a later question that indicates you answered a previous question incorrectly. If so, go back and change your earlier answer!

# Chapter 10

# Adding Street Cred: Specialty Certifications and Continuing Ed

Consider credentials the golden tickets to your medical billing and coding career. They give you credibility as a coder. In Chapter 7, I explain the basic certifications offered by the AAPC and AHIMA (the CPC, the CCA, and the CCS, for example). In this chapter, I introduce you to these organizations' specialty certifications.

Specialty certifications indicate extensive knowledge in particular areas of coding. These certifications are obtained by taking exams specific to the certifying organizations. Yet so many specialty certifications are available that picking one can seem overwhelming, but it really isn't that hard: Just pick what best bolsters your bona fides as a coder.

Beyond the specialty certifications are continuing education opportunities that keep you abreast of what's going on in your field. This chapter has the details.

## Getting Familiar with Your Specialty Certification Options

Both the AAPC (formerly the American Academy of Professional Coders) and the American Health Information Management Association (AHIMA) offer specialty certifications that can you can achieve as you develop your career. Earning a specialty certification shows an employer that you're striving to become an expert in your profession and an asset to the position. Adding specialty certifications also makes you highly marketable in your field.

Other organizations offer certifications, as well. These include the Board of Medical Specialty Coding and Compliance (BMSC) and the Professional Association of Healthcare Coding Specialists (PAHCS) among others. Note that neither of these have the history of the AAPC or AHIMA, but they are options. The BMSC, for example, was created to offer people who already have basic certification a way to credential their specialty knowledge. It's not an organization that a novice would normally benefit from.

Certifications are only as credible as the organization that gives them. Do your homework to find the most appropriate and reputable for your situation.

## AAPC trademarked certifications

The AAPC offers several trademarked certifications. These specialty certifications do not require you to get a Certified Professional Coder (CPC) certification (refer to Chapter 7), although each requires continuing education specific to the defined specialty. Thorough knowledge of medical terminology, anatomy, and physiology is also a must. These certifications, listed in Table 10-1, are beneficial to those already working in a medical office.

| Table 10-1 | Trademark AAPC Certifications |
|---|---|
| *Certification* | *Related Skills and Competencies* |
| Certified Ambulatory Surgery Center Coder (CASCC) | Ability to read and assign the correct codes and modifiers to procedures performed in an ambulatory surgery center (ASC); understanding rules for ASC reimbursement, including the multiple procedure discount coding for discontinued procedures |
| Certified Anesthesia and Pain Management Coder (CANPC) | Proficiency in selecting the highest based anesthesia CPT code for surgical cases and assigning the appropriate American Society of Anesthesiologist (ASA) codes; correctly using anesthesia modifiers and determining base units for cases; having a good grasp of procedures performed by physicians specializing in physical medicine, rehab and pain management |

| Certification | Related Skills and Competencies |
|---|---|
| Certified Cardiology Coder (CCC) | Proficiency in coding surgical procedures, including heart catheterization, coronary interventions, and vascular procedures, that are performed by cardiologists |
| Certified Chiropractic Professional Coder (CCPC) | Proficiency in coding procedures performed by licensed chiropractors |
| Certified Emergency Department Coder (CEDC) | Proficiency in coding surgical procedures performed by emergency department physicians; awareness of evaluation and management guidelines and time-based code protocol |
| Certified ENT Coder (CENTC) | Proficiency in coding ENT (ear, nose, throat) procedures, as well as determining appropriate evaluation and management codes by reading office notes and operative reports (which may document surgical procedures performed by otolaryngologists) |
| Certified Evaluation and Management Coder (CEMC) | Expertise in assigning the correct evaluation and management codes by identifying the level of visit based on the three key components of medical decision making |
| Certified Family Practice Coder (CFPC) | Expertise in determining the correct kind of evaluation and management codes to capture the level of visit; proficiency in coding minor surgical and ancillary procedures that a family practitioner may perform; full understanding of relative value unit (RVU) sequencing |
| Certified Gastroenterology Coder (CGIC) | Proficiency in coding procedures performed by gastroenterologists; determining evaluation and management codes |
| Certified General Surgery Coder (CGSC) | Proficiency in coding surgical procedures performed by general surgeons; knowledgeable in global periods and RVU sequencing |

*(continued)*

**Table 10-1 *(continued)***

| Certification | Related Skills and Competencies |
|---|---|
| Certified Hematology and Oncology Coder (CHONC) | Proficiency in coding surgical and therapeutic procedures performed by hematologists, oncologists, and members of their staff |
| Certified Internal Medicine Coder (CIMC) | Proficiency in determining billable procedures based on physician office notes, including office procedures (injections, vaccinations, and so on) and minor surgical procedures (such as joint injections) |
| Certified Interventional Radiology Cardiovascular Coder (CIRCCO) | Expertise in interventional radiology and cardiovascular coding; proficiency in coding cardio-related items (like diagnostic angiography), cardiac catheterizations, and nonvascular procedures |
| Certified Obstetrical Gynecology Coder (COBGC) | Proficiency in coding obstetric services and surgical procedures normally performed by OB/GYNs |
| Certified Pediatric Coder (CPEDC) | Proficiency in coding office procedures and surgical procedures performed by pediatricians, as well as determining correct evaluation and management codes based on office notes |
| Certified Plastics and Reconstructive Surgery Coder (CPRC) | Expertise in coding surgical procedures performed by plastic and reconstructive surgeons, as well as the ability to identify procedures considered cosmetic |
| Certified Professional Coder in Dermatology (CPCD) | Proficiency in coding surgical procedures (including various types of lesion excisions) performed by dermatologists |
| Certified Professional Compliance Officer (CPCO) | Proficiency in understanding the requirements necessary to develop and implement a compliance protocol for a medical office |

| Certification | Related Skills and Competencies |
|---|---|
| Certified Professional Medical Auditor (CPMA) | Proficiency in coding and documentation guidelines; being able to offer advice to improve a facility's or practice's revenue cycle; possessing advanced knowledge of medical documentation, fraud, and abuse as well as a familiarity with penalties for violations based on government regulations |
| Certified Rheumatology Coder (CRHC) | Proficiency with evaluation and management codes and surgical procedures performed by rheumatologists |
| Certified Urology Coder (CUC) | Expertise in coding office and surgical procedures performed by urologists |

# Specialty AHIMA certifications

Much like its kissing cousin, the AAPC, AHIMA offers several types of specialty certifications. It's a veritable alphabet soup of acronyms and designations, but fear not: I explain them all in the following sections.

## Registered Health Information Administrator (RHIA)

As a Registered Health Information Administrator (RHIA), you are an expert in managing medical records, including patient information and computer systems. You also have in-depth knowledge of ethical and legal requirements and standards with regard to the healthcare industry.

To be eligible for this certification, you must

✔ Have completed an accredited Health Informatics and Information Management (HIIM) program or have graduated from an HIIM program approved by a foreign association with which AHIMA has a reciprocity agreement.

✔ Have a degree from a Commission on Accreditation for Health Informatics and Information Management (CAHIIM) program. A directory of these programs is available on the CAHIIM website (www.cahiim.org). CAHIIM is the organization that accredits associate and bachelor's and master's degree programs in health information management.

# HIIM? HIIM who?

Health Informatics and Information Management (HIIM) deals with just about everything associated with the information created, disseminated, and shared by the healthcare industry, soup to nuts. From local information technology and interpersonal digital relations between physicians, clinics, and hospitals to coding information for Medicare and Medicaid, information management plays a role in how all the healthcare pieces work together. Making sure that patient data is managed with the utmost integrity is paramount, and it is part and parcel of an ongoing national effort to reduce medical errors and high costs for both physician and patient.

A strong foundation in HIIM is important for anyone wanting to earn certification in a related field. The impending total shift to electronic health records promises a secure future for anyone involved in the health information and informatics industry, so getting a degree in HIIM is going to be a win-win.

To talk nuts and bolts, the HIIM-related degree preps you for all sorts of career opportunities. For example, according to the University of Tennessee's Health Science Center, its Master of HIIM degree prepares you for careers in healthcare administration, data security oversight, strategic and operational information resource planning, clinical data analysis, clinical classification systems and support systems, information systems development, and even electronic health records implementation and management. In short, the HIIM world is your oyster. Don't wait — get on the HIIM bus ASAP.

## Registered Health Information Technician (RHIT)

As a Registered Health Information Technician (RHIT), you are certified to ensure completion and accuracy of medical records, including proper entry into computer systems. You may also specialize in coding medical records.

This certification is often held in combination with a bachelor's degree. To be eligible, you must have completed an accredited HIIM program (accreditation is through the Commission on Accreditation for Health Informatics and Information Management Education) or have graduated from a HIIM program approved by a foreign association with which AHIMA has a reciprocity agreement.

## Certified Health Data Analyst (CHDA)

To achieve the Certified Health Data Analyst (CHDA) certification level, you must demonstrate expertise in health data analysis. As the healthcare industry becomes more data driven and the use of electronic medical records continues to increase, practitioners will need individuals who can focus on the future of their practices and develop strategies to stay viable. To be eligible for this certification, you must have either of the following:

✔ A bachelor's degree or higher and a minimum of five years of healthcare data experience

✔ A RHIA credential and a minimum of one year of experience in health-care data

### Certified in Healthcare Privacy and Security (CHPS)

The Certified in Healthcare Privacy and Security (CHPS) certification identi-fies you as competent in protecting privacy and security programs in all types of healthcare information management. To be eligible for this certifica-tion, you must have any of the following:

✔ A bachelor's degree with a minimum of four years of experience in healthcare management

✔ A master's degree (or equivalent) with a minimum of two years of expe-rience in healthcare management

✔ A HIIM credential of RHIT or RHIA with a bachelor's degree or higher and a minimum of two years of healthcare management experience

## The best of the rest

The AAPC and AHIMA aren't the only games in town. Although they are per-haps the most well-known, you may discover that your professional goals would be better met by getting certified by another organization or by adding certifications from other organizations on to your AAPC or AHIMA certifica-tions. In the following sections, I discuss two reputable certifying organiza-tions: the Board of Medical Specialty Coding and Compliance (BMSC) and the Professional Association of Healthcare Coding Specialists (PAHCS).

### Board of Medical Specialty Coding and Compliance (BMSC)

BMSC is a lesser-known provider of specialty medical coding certifications and training for coders, compliance officers, and clinicians. BMSC certifica-tions encompass those who work in physician offices, as well as home health-care professionals.

Because the levels of education required in coding and compliance build from one certification level to another, BMSC certification helps coders and other professionals move up the career ladder.

The BMSC's certifications include the following:

✔ **Specialty Coding Professional (SCP) and Advanced Coding Specialist (ACS),** both of which offer specialty certification in numerous areas

✔ **Certified Compliance Professional-Physician (CCP-P),** a certification for compliance professionals in physician offices

- ✔ **Home Care Coding Specialist-Diagnosis (HCS-D)** for home care coders with experience in that area

- ✔ **Home Care Clinical Specialist-OASIS (HCS-O)** for home healthcare clinicians

All the BMSC certifications are directed to those who already have experience in the specified areas. Recertification requires taking an exam every two years and renewing your membership annually.

### Professional Association of Healthcare Coding Specialists (PAHCS)

PAHCS is a support organization that functions as a communication network for members. This organization serves primarily as a support system for coders working in a medical practice, but membership is open to all coding professionals.

Certification by this organization involves submitting an application and completing a written examination that shows proficiency within the ambulatory healthcare delivery system. If you've been certified by other organizations, you may receive PAHCS certification by showing proof of current certification and paying a membership fee and a processing fee.

# Building on Your Cred with Continuing Education

Regardless of which certification(s) you choose, you've got to participate in some continuing education to maintain it. The healthcare industry is constantly evolving. Codes change. Rules change. Medicare policies change. A claim form that's been used for several years is replaced. Every year, diagnosis codes and new CPT codes are added while older codes are retired. Soon you'll have to consider the change to ICD-10. Continuing education keeps you up to date on all the pertinent changes.

## Adding up the continuing ed units (CEUs)

The number of continuing education units (CEUs) you need varies based on the type of certification(s) you have. Each specialty certification requires units in that specialty in addition to the basic certification requirements. Table 10-2 shows the current CEU requirements for AAPC certifications.

| Table 10-2 | AAPC CEU Requirements |
|---|---|
| *Number of Certifications* | *CEUs Required* |
| 1 certification | 36 CEUs every two years (see note) |
| 2 certifications | 48 CEUs every two years with specialty-specific requirements (see note) |
| 3 certifications | 60 CEUs, with specialty-specific requirements (see note) |
| 4 certifications | 72 CEUs every two years (see note) |
| 5+ certifications | 80 CEUs every two years, with specialty-specific certification requirements (see note) |

**Note:** *The CIRCC, CPMA, and CPCO certifications (mentioned earlier in this chapter) require that at least 24 of the CEUs in a two-year period be credential-specific.*

Ask your credentialing organization about how many CEUs are needed for each credential before you decide which program to go with. Knowing how much time is involved later may help you make the wisest decision now.

AHIMA continuing education requirements differ slightly. They require completion of CEUs in addition to mandatory annual coding self-assessments (available through AHIMA). The level of certification dictates the number of CEUs required per two-year cycle: CCA, CCS, and CCS-P require 20 CEUs in addition to two self-assessments per cycle. RHIA, CHDA, CHP, and CHS each require 30 CEUs. The RHIT requirement is 20 CEUs.

Multiple AHIMA certifications require different numbers of CEUs, depending on the individual certifications. You can find out about specific requirements on the AHIMA website (www.ahima.org).

## Earning the units you need

You earn CEUs by attending workshops, professional boot camps, and webinars and by taking quizzes linked to professional articles in coding magazines or technical publications.

The credentialing organization determines the number of CEUs the various activities offer after evaluating the educational content of a program. The number of CEUs associated with an activity normally coincides with that activity's time commitment. One hour equals one CEU. Exceptions are meetings and workshops. Often, organization meetings earn you ½ or 1 CEU, even though these activities last two or more hours. (Time is counted for the time spent in actual learning, not in coffee or lunch breaks and definitely not for meeting with vendors to grab your take-home goodies!)

Make sure your credentialing organization has approved the activity you want to use as a CEU. Approved articles, quizzes, meetings, webinars, and so on display the organization's approval seal, along with the number of CEUs you can earn.

Each time you earn a CEU, you receive a certificate that has an index number that you register with the AAPC. This number verifies that the CEU is authentic. Go to AAPC's online CEU tracker (available to members) and enter the index number into the tracker. Be sure to hold on to the paper copies of your certificates, though. You'll need them in the event that you're randomly selected for a CEU audit.

## Finding free CEU resources

Some free CEU resources are available if you know where to look. Read on to find out more.

### Getting free AAPC units

Membership in the AAPC includes a subscription to the organization's magazine, *The Coding Edge*. Each month, the AAPC website includes an online quiz covering articles in that month's publication. Complete the quiz, and your CEU is automatically linked to your account. How's that for healthcare information management?

Other free resources may be local chapter opportunities or attendance at certain lectures. You can contact the AAPC directly to inquire about opportunity in your area.

### Getting free AHIMA units

AHIMA offers five recorded webinars that are related to its Program for Evaluating Payment Patterns, which is aimed at hospital management. Check out www.ahima.org/continuinged for links to the webinars, as well as audio resources, event and conference listings, and a host of other professional resources geared toward coders.

### Medicare's web-based training

Medicare offers web-based training, organized into a series of modules. The web modules offered by Uncle Sam are quite informative, and you can complete them at your own pace. These training exercises are relevant to current coding and processing issues, and Medicare updates them regularly, keeping you abreast of the latest developments and changes. After you complete the web training, you take an online quiz. Pass the quiz and earn a free CEU.

You need to enter these CEUs into your AAPC CEU tracker account yourself. If you are earning CEUs toward other organization certifications, you need to follow their protocol for submitting them. Check out `www.cms.gov/mln products/03_webbasedtraining.asp` for more information about this great resource.

## Getting the most bang for your buck with CEUs

You often need to earn CEUs on your own time (and your own dollar), in which case you want to make sure you're getting the most benefit for the cost. In the next sections, I offer advice on which activities provide a good cost-to-CEU ratio.

### Workshops

Attending a one day conference or workshop that offers 8 or 10 CEUs can be an economical use of your time, given that you need at minimum of 18 units each year. Attending a conference or workshop is a good idea especially if the meeting is relevant to your current position or to the position you hope to get.

Both the AAPC and AHIMA offer workshops that allow coders to not only earn CEUs but, most importantly, to also learn about updates to policies, procedures, and diagnosis codes. Attending these can be costly (check with your employer to see whether it will subsidize your attendance), but the price is often worth it. Compared to online learning or reading articles, attending a workshop gives you the opportunity to ask questions and network with the instructors and other attendees. Medicare also hosts training through a program called Provider Outreach and Education. The goal of this program is to educate providers and their staffs about fundamentals of Medicare, including policies, procedures, and changes to the Medicare program.

Medicare also offers numerous training opportunities: live training through seminars, teleconferences, and webinars; on-demand training through audio and audio-visual presentations including educational materials; and online training through the Medicare Learning Network, a web-based program that targets different provider types. These opportunities are usually free if you sign up in advance.

### Boot camps

Boot camps are learning-intensive workshops. They normally span a two- or three-day period and can supply you with a lot of CEUs. Check with the AAPC or AHIMA to find out about boot camps in your area.

### Paid subscriptions

A host of paid subscriptions target specialty areas from anesthesia to urology. Subscribers to these publications or websites normally have the opportunity to earn CEUs by completing online quizzes that cover current and past articles. The good thing about subscribing to these resources is that you can review them on your own schedule and as often as you like. The downside is that, if you need clarification, you have to write a letter or send an e-mail to the editor(s) and wait for the answer. If you tend to be impatient, you may want to keep some other resources at your disposal as well.

# Part IV

# Dealing with the Nitty-Gritty On-the-Job Details

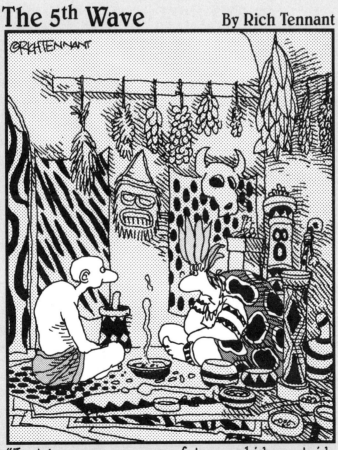

## The 5th Wave

By Rich Tennant

"Just leave your co-pay of two ox hides outside my tent, and we'll bill you for the rest."

# In this part . . .

Welcome to the grand tour of the day-to-day of medical billing and coding. This is the place where all the work you do to get educated and certified finally pays off. In this part, I walk you through the claim filing process: I explain all that goes into getting the claim out the door on time and accurately and offer tips and tricks for turning those codes into cash. Big money, after all, *is* the name of the billing and coding game, so you can rest assured that the chapters in this part give you the play-by-play details that let you win big for your clients.

# Chapter 11

# Processing a Run-of-the-Mill Claim: An Overview

. . . . . . . . . . . . . . . . . . . . . . . . . . . . . . . . . . . . . . . . . . . . . . . . . . . . .

. . . . . . . . . . . . . . . . . . . . . . . . . . . . . . . . . . . . . . . . . . . . . . . . . . . . .

**A**s a biller and coder, you perform magic daily by converting physician- or specialist-performed services into revenue. You perform this feat through the fine art of claims processing. *Claims processing* is the industry term that refers to the general process of submitting and following up on claims. Of course, you can break this general process down into particular tasks, like gathering the necessary demographic information from the patient, abstracting the codes themselves from the provider's documentation of the patient encounter, entering the codes into the billing software, and so on.

In this chapter, I outline the general claims submittal process from beginning to end to give you a solid foundation in how things work and who does what along the way. For detailed information on actually preparing a claim for submission, head to the other chapters in this part.

## The Perfect Billing Scenario

Although every billing scenario is a bit different, they all follow, to a large degree, the same general process. In this section, I explain what the ideal billing situation looks like. When everything goes according to plan and all the moving parts of the billing and coding process work as they should, you end up with a fully paid claim that doesn't require follow up on your part.

# Completing the initial paperwork

When you walk into the office of any healthcare provider, be it a family physician, a testing lab, or the emergency room, what's the first thing you do? You walk up to the desk and check in, of course. As a biller and coder, this initial interaction is the first step in the billing scenario.

During the check-in, a couple of things happen:

- ✔ **The patient completes a demographic form.** This form identifies the patient name, birthdate, address, and Social Security number or driver's license number. The form should also indicate who the policyholder of the insurance is and what that person's relationship is to the patient. If the policyholder is someone other than the patient, then the same information (name, birthdate, and so on) should be obtained about the policyholder, as well.

  Copy the patient's insurance card at each encounter, both front and back, when you request the demographic form.

- ✔ **You verify the patient's identity by asking for a government issued photo ID.** Thanks to a proliferation of insurance fraud and identity theft (thanks, technology!), you need to make sure that the patient who brings in an insurance card is actually the insured member.

  Using another individual's insurance coverage is fraud, and a provider who submits a claim that misrepresents an encounter is also committing fraud. So be alert and double-check the ID the patient hands you, because every provider is responsible for verifying patient identity and could be held liable for fraud committed in the provider's office.

- ✔ **You verify whether the patient needs a referral or a preauthorization.** To find out more about what these are and why you need to check them early, hop to the section "Covering Your Bases: Referrals and Preauthorization."

- ✔ **You verify benefits.** Here are some benefit-related questions to ask upfront:

  - **Is there a copay?** If so, the provider is normally expected to collect that amount up front.

  - **Is there any unmet deductible?** If the patient has an unmet deductible, the provider may want to ask for all or part of that up front.

  - **Is the patient out-of-network, and if so, what are his out-of-network benefits?**

- ✔ **You collect any copayments, deductibles, or co-insurance obligations.** If the provider encounter is a procedure to which a deductible or co-insurance obligation may be incurred, these amounts may also be collected up front.

## Getting the documentation about the patient encounter with the provider

After the initial paperwork is complete, the next step of the revenue cycle is the actual patient encounter with the service provider or physician.

Following the encounter, the provider documents the billable services. This documentation includes what was done, the reason the service was medically necessary, and any additional information that the physician feels is relevant to the patient's care. In the past, the charts were paper, and the documentation was usually handwritten. Today, providers are moving toward electronic health records. These records contain the same information which is much easier to read than handwriting.

## Entering the codes into the billing software

With the patient information gathered at check in and the provider documentation of the patient encounter, you have the information you need to enter the correct CPT and ICD-9 codes into the billing software. This is the general procedure:

1. **You enter the patient information into the billing software.**

   This information includes patient demographics, payer information, and financial guarantor information (see the section "Completing the initial paperwork").

   If the patient has two insurances, one is primary and one is secondary. Some patients may have more than two carriers. If so, you enter that information into the billing software, too, along with the order in which the insurance carriers should be billed.

2. **You abstract the billable codes based on what the physician documentation says.**

3. **You enter the information — the CPT (procedure) and ICD-9 (diagnosis) codes — into the appropriate claim form in the billing software.**

4. **You send the claim off.**

   In most cases, the claim is electronically uploaded to a medical clearinghouse to then be sent to the appropriate payer. In some cases, the claim is sent directly to the payer. To find out more about billing software, jump to the later section "Working with billing software."

Many carriers have claims submission portals on their websites that allow providers to submit claims directly. However, because the process can be time consuming (due to having individual websites for each carrier), this system isn't efficient for larger providers. Also, medical billing software and clearinghouse software provide code-editing services that help prevent claim rejections due to clerical coding errors — an advantage you miss if you submit claims directly.

To get the provider paid, you have to submit every single claim as obligated by the payer contract. Unfortunately, every payer seems to have different rules, and you'll encounter thousands of little billing and coding peculiarities unique to each payer — too many to mention here, in fact. The best way to find out about these rules and payer-specific peculiarities is to read the contract or call the payer relations line to verify submission requirements.

## Show me the money!

After the payer receives the claim, the payer reviews the claim to determine the following:

- ✔ Whether medical necessity has been met.
- ✔ Whether the claim is covered by the patient's plan.
- ✔ What the reimbursement allowance is. To determine this, the payer references the contract that may be in place with the service provider.

After the terms of the contract have been met, the claim will process and pay under the terms of the patient's plan.

What makes this scenario perfect? The patient is insured, the provider has a contract with either the payer or the network to which the payer belongs, and the claim is clean (that is, it can be processed using only the information provided, it contains no errors, and the correct contract is loaded into the payer claims software). The point? A lot of things impact how smoothly processing a claim goes.

# Delving into the Details: Contract Specifics

Every payer has its own policies and procedures manual, and as the coder, you need to be knowledgeable about individual payer requirements. The best place to find that payer information is in the contract. The contract also defines the levels of payment for each of the network providers. As a biller and coder, one of the most important parts of your job is understanding contracts and how they determine the amount of reimbursement the provider receives.

Normally, you have access to the payer contract: It will be programmed into your billing software. Ideally, the payer contracts are pre-loaded into the software, allowing you to view the contract on a network drive. If not, you can print a paper copy. As you read through the contract, you see that each set of policies contains subsets that apply to the various plans sponsored by the payer or that apply to the network that the payer participates in. Examples of subsets include the plan benefits available to HMO members versus the plan benefits available to PPO members.

## Who's contracting who?

In the case of contracts, the payers (insurance companies) are in charge. They offer various levels of coverage to their members. When contracting with the insurance company for employee group coverage, the patient's employer often selects the level of coverage it will offer its employees. In this case, the insurance company is *underwriting* the plan, which means that the employer pays the insurer, who is then responsible for paying the covered services within the confines of the contract.

Some employers find that underwriting their own policies is more cost effective. In that case, the employer may contract with a network, or third party administrator, for pricing of claims, but the actual payment comes from the employer. Check out Chapter 6 for more information about third party administrators.

The insurance company or network also contracts with healthcare providers to participate within the network. Here's the idea: The company directs patients to providers in its network, thus increasing the number of patients (and payments) these providers get. In return, the providers help keep the payer costs under control by limiting the amount of reimbursement they receive for each encounter. By staying within the payer network, the patient saves the insurance company or employer money while still receiving quality healthcare.

Whenever possible, providers try to participate in the plans or networks that underwrite the majority of the local population (that's a cost savings).

## Looking at standard contracts

Many payers or networks have standardized contracts that they offer to healthcare providers. A well-defined contract does the following:

✔ Defines the number of days after the encounter that the provider has to submit the claim. This is called *timely filing*.

✔ Specifies how many days after receipt of the claim the payer has to make payment. Some states have prompt claim pay laws, and it's important to know what each state requires. If the payer is not compliant with either the contract or state laws, penalties are usually applied in the form of interest that compounds daily.

✔ Specifies which of the payer plans are included, the frequency of services that it will cover (for certain procedures), and the type of claim that is to be submitted by the provider.

✔ Identifies special circumstances that may affect either the provider or the payer, such as

- How unlisted procedures are to be reimbursed (these procedures end in "99" and are usually worded in a way that states "other unspecified procedure")

    Medicare and some other government payers will not pay unlisted procedures. Other commercial payers simply deny payment unless the provider's contract specifically obligates it.

- The appeals process

- Procedures that are carved out of the fee schedule to be paid a set amount (see the next section for more on carve-outs)

- The number of procedures that the payer will pay per encounter

- The multiple procedure discount (the discount applied to procedures that are paid in addition to the initial procedure)

✔ Identifies cost intensive supplies or procedures that may need to be paid. This may include such items as implants, screws, anchors, plates, rods, and so on.

✔ Carves out payment for intensive services or procedures at 65 percent of billed charges.

Even though they're standardized, every payer contract is different in one way or another. Make sure you read each contract carefully and familiarize yourself with each set of payer circumstances.

## Understanding reimbursement rates and carve-outs

As I explain in the preceding section, despite their differences, contracts tend to be fairly boilerplate. These contracts are similar to Medicare's fee schedule, and they may be based on that schedule. They may pay 110 percent or

125 percent of what Medicare allows. They may even pay less than Medicare allows, which sometimes happens with large networks or payers who have so many insured members that providers risk financial disaster by not participating. (In such a case, providers can't really afford to not participate because the number of patients in the practice will fall drastically.)

Providers who want to become part of a specific network first identify which services they expect to provide and how much they need to be paid to be profitable within the network. The providers also factor in all overhead costs (rent, utilities, staff, commodities, and salary) associated with each type of service. They also may identify specific services that they'd like to be carve-outs of the contract.

A *contracted carve-out* is a special clause in the contract that stipulates a different payment rate from the normal rate for a specified procedural code. These carve-outs are important parts of provider contracts. Although they should result in a profit for the provider, they often delay correct claims processing because they require special handling by the payer. To put it simply, the carve-out isn't a simple line item that the payer's computerized processing system can automatically assign payment for; instead it's a clause that requires additional care when coding *and* paying.

# Covering Your Bases: Referrals and Preauthorization

Contracted providers should know what services each payer does and doesn't cover. Some payers, for example, don't pay for procedures that are considered investigative or experimental; others don't pay for unlisted procedures. Medicare doesn't pay for any procedure that is unlisted, and many payers follow Medicare guidelines as a matter of course.

That's why, prior to a patient encounter, you must check the patient's plan benefits in addition to the provider contract. Doing so lets you identify potential reimbursement issues in advance and know what, if any, special protocol needs to be followed. Two of the more common scenarios you'll encounter involve checking referrals and securing preauthorization.

## Checking for referrals

If the patient's plan requires a referral, make sure a referral was given. Check in the record to ensure that the referral is noted (it is usually an alphanumeric entry that must be included on the claim). For certain HMO plans, the primary care physician submits the referral to the payer prior to the specialist encounter; then, when the payer receives the claim, the payer knows that the visit was authorized.

Although many plans place the responsibility for obtaining the referral on the patient, it's in the best interest of both the patient and the provider for you to assist in this endeavor. The provider is the professional and in the best position to understand what steps are necessary to treat the patient.

## Dealing with prior authorization

*Prior authorization* (also known as *preauthorization*) is the process of getting an agreement from the payer to cover specific services before the service is performed. Normally, a payer that authorizes a service prior to an encounter assigns an authorization number that you need to include on the claim when you submit it for payment.

### Getting the correct CPT code beforehand

The key to a solid preauthorization is to provide the correct CPT code. The challenge is that you have to determine the correct procedural code before the service has been provided (and documented) — an often difficult task.

To determine the correct code, check with the physician to find out what she anticipates doing. Make sure you get all possible scenarios; otherwise, you run the risk that a procedure that was performed won't be covered. For example, if the doctor has scheduled a biopsy (which may not need prior authorization) but then actually excises a lesion (which probably does need prior authorization), the claim for the excision will be denied. What's a coder to do? Authorize the excision! It's better to authorize treatment not rendered than to be denied payment for no authorization. No penalty is incurred when a procedure has been authorized but is not completed, so err on the side of preauthorization.

In rare cases, the patient coverage is unavailable prior to an encounter. This scenario most often occurs in emergency situations, due to an accident or sudden illness that develops during the night or on weekends. When this happens, the servicing provider must contact the payer as soon as possible and secure the necessary authorizations.

Although you are the coder in charge of assigning the appropriate codes, the burden of obtaining necessary authorizations is largely on the provider, because it's the provider who'll be denied payment as expected. Getting preauthorization takes only a few minutes, and it can save countless hours on the back end trying to chase claim payments. Preauthorization also results in faster claims processing and prompt payments.

### When you don't get the necessary preauthorization

Who gets stuck with footing the bill when preauthorizations don't pan out? It depends. The determination as to who is responsible is often defined by the patient's insurance plan. If the plan benefits outline specific services that are not covered and the patient seeks those services, the responsibility for payment falls to the patient. On the other hand, if a provider fails to authorize treatment prior to providing services to a patient and payment is denied by the insurance company, then the provider may be obligated to absorb the cost of treatment, and no payment is due from the patient.

Many payers don't issue retro authorizations, even when the failure to get preauthorization was a mistake. Some may overturn a denial on appeal, but they're under no obligation to make payment if the proper process was not followed.

Some payers may assign full financial responsibility for a procedure that didn't get the necessary preauthorization to the patient. In this case, the provider has to make a decision about whether to pursue collecting the payment from the patient. Some swallow the loss. Others send the unpaid bill to the patient, but doing so is bad business. Patients are both unaware of the process and not in any sort of position to guess what CPT code should be submitted to the insurance company. This is yet another reason to do your homework as a coder and make sure those preauthorizations are going to go through.

Occasionally you run into a situation in which the patient's coverage was verified prior to services, and the patient's employer terminates benefits retroactively. This usually happens when there is a termination of employment that is challenged in court or when an employer learns that a covered employee was in violation of his or her contract during employment. In these very unfortunate situations, the patient is responsible for the medical fees, but collecting the debt can be quite difficult.

# Tracking Your Claim from Submission to Payment

As you read earlier, the claims process begins when you enter the CPT and ICD-9 codes into the billing software, but it certainly doesn't end there. Your claim will take a (potentially arduous) journey on the path to payment. In the following sections, I explain the stops and possible perils along the way, from billing software to the clearinghouses to the payer.

Of course, not all submissions have happy endings; they get stuck along the way. In that case, you need to file an appeal. For details on that process, head to the section "Appealing to the Masses: Filing an Appeal with the Payer."

## Working with billing software

Everything that happens in the claims process is reliant on the software you use to code. Consider this software the backbone of what you do. It prepares the claim to be submitted to the claims clearinghouse (covered in the next section).

### Features of the software

Many different types of billing software are available, but they all allow you to enter the procedure codes and diagnosis codes, as well as the provider's fee for each code, the patient's insurance information (policy number and group number), and the payer's address. The software also links each payer to a specific payer ID.

Most of the newer versions of billing software are compatible with electronic medical records (EMRs), in which case the billing modules of the software are included with the clinical modules of the patient's record. What this means is that the clinical staff clinical enters the clinical information and provides additional documentation of medical necessity.

Here are some other features you may encounter:

- ✔ Some offices use billing software that links into their electronic medical records, while other offices have encounter-specific information (encounter times, names of clinical staff involved in the encounter, and so on) stored in the billing software. This information is useful for inventory purposes, to determine the cost of each patient's care, and in the event of any legal inquiries.

- ✔ Some offices have security edits in place that allow access to various parts of this software based on the employee's need to know or clearance. Access to the patient's personal history, for example, may not be viewable by the billing staff, and access to patient demographic information, such as Social Security number, may not be viewable by the charge-nurse.

Numerous types of billing software systems are available, and the one you use depends on the provider's needs and budget, but the primary purpose of all billing software is to serve as a platform to prepare the claim to begin its journey, which ends when the provider receives payment from the insurance company or other payer.

### *Making sure the correct contract is loaded into the billing software*

Normally, payer contracts are already loaded into the office billing software so that, when you enter information, the software automatically links each procedure to the appropriate payment obligated by the payer contract.

Having the correct contract loaded saves time because it facilitates payment posting on the back end of the claim. Here's why: When the insurance company makes a payment, the payment is posted to each patient account. The person responsible for posting payments is referred to as the *payment poster.* If the contract isn't loaded correctly, the payment poster must verify each payment to make sure that it's correct.

In small companies, the payment poster may be the office manager or other front office associate. Larger companies, including most billing companies, have employees whose job is limited to just posting payments to the correct accounts.

## From provider to clearinghouse

Companies that serve as intermediaries who forward claims information from healthcare providers to insurance payers are known as *clearinghouses.* In what is called *claims scrubbing,* clearinghouses check the claim for errors and verify that it is compatible with the payer software. The clearinghouse also checks to make sure that the procedural and diagnosis codes being submitted are valid and that each procedure code is appropriate for the diagnosis code submitted with it. The claim scrubbing edit helps prevent time-consuming processing errors.

Each provider chooses which clearinghouse it wants to use for submitting claims. Most clearinghouse companies charge the providers for each claim submitted, and they also charge an additional fee to send a paper claim to a certain payer.

Clearinghouses may submit claims directly to the payers, or they may have to send a claim through other clearinghouse sites before reaching the payer(s). The claims may go through other clearinghouses for the following reasons:

✔ **The provider billing software isn't compatible with the payer processing software, and the information needs to be reformatted prior to being sent to the payer.** Because of the potential difficulties caused by incompatible software, clearinghouses require an initial enrollment period prior to sending claims for the first time. During the enrollment period, which can take up to four weeks, the clearinghouse tests the compatibility between the provider software and the payer software.

Providers need to be mindful of this process so that their claims are not delayed. When using a new clearinghouse, verify the enrollment process before you actually need to submit live claims. (Also check the clearinghouses payer list. You want to choose a clearinghouse that already has a relationship with your payers.)

✔ **The payer isn't enrolled in the same clearinghouse the provider uses.** The provider pays the clearinghouse, and the insurance companies pay the clearinghouse. Each payer is identified by its clearinghouse *electronic data interchange* (EDI) number. This number serves as the payer's "address," or identifier, and it tells the clearinghouse which payer to send the claim to. If the payer isn't enrolled in the same clearinghouse as the provider, the claim is sent to a clearinghouse that the payer is enrolled with. Take a look at a couple of examples.

- **Example 1:** Provider Smith uses ABC billing software. Provider Smith then enrolls with XYZ clearinghouse. ABC software sends the claims entered into it to XYZ clearinghouse. Payer Gold is enrolled with the same XYZ clearinghouse. So XYZ receives Provider Smith's claims and sends them directly to Payer Gold. This is a simple exchange, and the claim is paid fairly quickly.

- **Example 2:** Provider Smith uses ABC billing software and enrolls with XYZ clearinghouse. Payer Gold isn't enrolled with XYZ clearinghouse; it's enrolled with JKL clearinghouse. So XYZ clearinghouse must send the claims to JKL clearinghouse before they can be sent to Payer Gold. This exchange takes longer to get the claim from the provider to the payer and may delay payment.

Obviously, if a clearinghouse has to send a claim to other clearinghouses, the claims process takes longer. In addition, exchanges like this can perpetuate, with your claims going every which way before reaching the intended payer. And every time the claim is transferred, the chances of it being stalled or lost increases. And round and round you go! To avoid this carousel of billing chaos, you need to know where the claims are going after they leave the provider.

If you are enrolled with a clearinghouse that seems to always send the claims to other clearinghouses, shopping around may be wise. Enrolling with a larger entity may cost a little more, but doing so is usually worthwhile if it gets the payment in sooner.

## *. . . And on to the payer*

After making its way through the clearinghouse, the claim finally ends up with the payer. The payer is responsible for paying the provider for services rendered to its client, the patient. Refer to Chapter 6 for information about the various payers.

### How claims are processed

The payer enters the claim into its processing software. What happens next depends on the claim. Claims that are compliant with the provider contract and patient's plan guidelines are usually paid promptly.

Claims that involve high dollar amounts or that need supporting documentation usually require *manual processing*. Unlike most claims, which are processed by computers, claims requiring manual processing need to be reviewed by a human. In addition to simply looking at the procedures, the payer reviews the diagnosis and other applicable documentation. For example, if the provider contract includes a carve-out for, say, implants (refer to the earlier section "Understanding reimbursement rates and carve-outs"), then the payer needs to see the invoice(s) and calculate the correct payment for that line. Or if a provider has billed an unlisted code and the contract allows payment for this code, then the payer may need to review additional information, such as an operative report, to determine which procedure the unlisted code represents. As you may guess, manual claims processing takes longer.

Each state has an insurance department or commissioner, and any commercial payers who violate state prompt pay laws or contractually obligated payment timelines may be reported to the appropriate official. When this happens, the department investigates the complaint and may take action either by serving notice to the payer that payment must be made immediately or, if deemed appropriate, revoking or suspending the payer's license to do business in that particular state. Keep in mind, however, that, even though payers are obligated by contracts to pay claims within a specific time period, that obligation is not enforceable if the provider doesn't submit the claims correctly or completely.

### Understanding claims matching

To pay for services rendered, the payer relies on the claims to be correct and truthful, often using a method called *claims matching*. When specific services are performed, several providers submit claims for the same patient. Here's an example: Say that a patient has a surgery. The surgeon submits a claim; the hospital or facility submits a claim; and the anesthesiologist submits a claim. Each claim is slightly different, of course, because each provider rendered a different service, but the surgeon's bill, the anesthesiologist's bill, and the facility's bill should match — that is, the same procedural codes should be on all three claims.

If you are a facility coder, you are actually breaking compliance rules if you call the physician coder to ask what he or she submitted. Stick to the coding. Both claims are based on the physician documentation, and if you follow coding protocol, the claims should match pretty well.

## Working out the Workers' Comp claim details

Each state has its own guidelines for Workers' Compensation claim payments. Some states have fee schedules; others don't. In states that have Workers' Compensation fee schedules, these fee schedules function the same as a provider contract; the claim processes according to the fee schedule. If the provider treats a Workers' Comp patient, the payment guidelines that apply are those where the patient's employer filed the claim, not where the provider is.

Check out this example. Patient Bob works for a company that is headquartered in Kentucky. Bob lives in Illinois (which has a Workers' Compensation state fee schedule) but has surgery in Missouri (which has no Workers' Compensation fee schedule). The Kentucky employer files the claim with its carrier in Kentucky, and the Missouri provider is obligated by the payment guidelines of Kentucky.

Therefore, if you're coding the payment for a Workers' Compensation claim settlement, educate yourself and possibly your employer about the Workers' Comp laws of the state where the claim was filed. Most states have this information on their websites. You can also obtain the necessary information by calling the State Department of Injured Workers.

If the state-legislated payment rules are violated and a commercial payer (refer to Chapter 6) sends incorrect payment, then the provider has grounds to file an appeal, and it's your job as the coder to appeal, appeal, and appeal again until your provider has been paid correctly. If no contract or pre-payment agreement exists, then the provider is under no obligation to accept the payment as full claim settlement. Bottom line: Know before you file.

If the bills don't match, the payer may request supporting documentation from any or all providers. In addition, if the surgeon and facility each bill for a completely different body part than that submitted on the anesthesia claim, an inquiry will likely occur. (*Note:* Some payers won't pay for facility charges or the anesthesia charges until after they've reviewed the surgeon's bill.)

Working together with other providers gets claims paid faster. And that should always be your goal: coding correctly and efficiently to secure accurate and prompt payment for your provider. If additional information is requested from a payer, promptly provide it. Failure to cooperate delays not only your claim but all related claims as well.

## Scoring the payment or going into negotiation

If the provider and payer have a contract in effect on the date the service was rendered and if the claim moved through the process as it should, the payment that the payer issues to the provider should be correct. If the payer and provider don't have a contract, the payer may send the claim to be priced by a third party in a process known as *negotiation*.

Some payers use third-party pricing companies to negotiate pricing for out-of-network claims. These companies serve as intermediaries in the negotiations between payer and provider. The intermediary contacts the provider and offers a negotiated settlement amount that is specific to an individual claim. Normally, this settlement offer also includes a prompt payment clause. After the provider signs the settlement, the payer sends the agreed upon payment. (You can read more about third-party administrators in Chapter 6.)

In a negotiation, the intermediary may do the following:

✓ **Arbitrarily price a claim and state that the pricing is "usual and customary" based on the geographical area where the services were provided:** These claims are often under priced, so be prepared to challenge the pricing.

✓ **Submit a settlement request to the provider:** These settlement agreements normally obligate a discounted payment to be sent within a specified time, usually 10 days or less.

These negotiation attempts are just that — attempts. The provider isn't obligated to accept the offer. In fact, providers should counter any initial offer they receive from a payer in these circumstances:

✓ **When a contract exists between provider and payer:** If the claim doesn't pay as specified by the contract, you should immediately notify the payer of the issue. Often, you can simply send the claim back with a notation explaining how the claim should have processed.

✓ **When no contract exists between payer and provider:** In this situation, the payer isn't entitled to a discount, even though the payer looks for a discount in most cases. If the provider hasn't accepted a pre-payment price reduction but the payer takes one, immediately notify the payer *in writing* that the payment is not acceptable. This written notice, sent upon receipt of an under-paid claim settlement, is known as a *claim appeal*. The important part of the appeal is to know the payment rules and stand firm on them. I go into more detail on appeals in the next section.

# Appealing to the Masses: Filing an Appeal with the Payer

If something goes haywire during the claims process and your provider doesn't get paid or doesn't receive the amount contracted, you need to file an appeal with the payer. Another point you may have to appeal is violation of prompt pay statutes.

## Big Brother is watching

Each state has a Department of Insurance that is responsible for making sure that insurance companies operating within the state follow the state's insurance laws. These laws are in place to protect citizens from exploitation or deception. Examples of problems that can get an insurance company in trouble with the insurance commissioner include selling policies to individuals but not paying claims, for example. You can locate the Department of Insurance for each state through the individual state's website.

Prompt pay statutes define how long a payer has to pay a claim after having received it. The prompt pay statutes are different in each state, so make sure you know the statute that applies to your provider. If the payer doesn't pay within the legislated time-frame, the statute usually obligates additional payment of interest, which accrues on each claim. Often, this accrual is per day.

If the payer delays or stalls payment, interest is due. Because the interest amount is usually small, providers often overlook it. Don't. Enforcing the prompt payment rules keeps payers accountable. Plus, if the situation were reversed, don't think for one minute that the payer(s) would not enforce the interest penalty.

When you file an appeal, make sure you base the appeal on facts. The phrase "It's not fair!" isn't sufficient grounds for appeal — but, of course, you already know that. If a contract exists between payer and provider, you need to quote the verbiage of the contract in the appeal. If the payer is refusing to honor a negotiated agreement, you refer to the agreement. If the payer still refuses to settle the matter to your satisfaction, then you may need to take the issue to the state insurance commissioner, an attorney who specializes in this area of the law, or the Department of Labor.

For detailed information on how to file an appeal (as well as how to resolve disputes), head to Chapter 14.

Remember the two golden rules of appealing a claim, and you'll be just fine in the coding world: First, keep impeccable documentation of every interaction you have with a payer. The paper trail you create might serve you well later when questions arise about the claims you process. And second, always, always keep your cool, on the phone and in writing. Think Dragnet style — just the facts, ma'am!

# Chapter 12

# Honing In on How to Prepare an Error-free Claim

***

### In This Chapter

▶ Entering the correct codes and modifiers

▶ Ensuring all billable codes are included

▶ Seeking clarification when the documentation is unclear

▶ Double-checking your work

***

*I*s any day better than payday? Personally, I think not. And I'm betting providers don't think so, either. That's why they hired you: to make sure all of the coding is right-on so they get paid right away. Let's face it: Money talks. As the coder, you're the one who converts the healthcare provider's work into revenue. The more accurate the coding, the better the revenue.

Your goal as a biller/coder is to make sure every encounter is documented properly. The codes must accurately represent the work performed. If you under code, for example, you're leaving money on the table: work was done, but you didn't request the fair payment. Similarly, if you submit codes that the documentation doesn't support or you unbundle procedures for the purpose of extra payment, you're committing what is known as fraudulent billing.

Your goal, then, is to make sure that you bill for every service for which your provider is entitled to be reimbursed. To do that properly, you need to know which services merit separate reimbursement (and which ones don't), how to gather the information you need to abstract the codes from the documentation, and what to check to make sure everything has been accurately represented. In this chapter, I tell you how to do all those things.

## Assigning CPT Codes

To get your provider paid, you've got to start somewhere, and that somewhere can be found by looking no further than the procedure codes (CPT codes) you submit on each claim. The more accurately you assign these codes, the more money the payer sends to the provider. But the earning potential of each claim depends on much more than just assigning codes and crossing your fingers. Instead, your coding must be accurate, without *under-coding* (leaving billable codes off of the claim) or *up-coding* (submitting codes that are not supported by the medical record), both of which can be considered fraudulent billing.

The magical little codes that help you turn patient encounters into cash for your provider are the most powerful part of each claim you code. They help prove to a payer that a medical product or service should be paid for.

## The lowdown on CPT codes and fee schedules

Each payer assigns a specific dollar amount to each CPT code; this lets the payer know how much to pay for the service rendered. Put all the codes and all their associated fees in a list, and you have a fee schedule.

Medical fee schedules are built from CPT codes that are often either priced individually or categorized into tiers:

- ✓ **Fee schedules with individual pricing:** Medicare and other payers, such as Tricare, price codes individually, and their fee schedules list each individual code and the payment assigned to that code.

- ✓ **Fee schedules with categorized pricing:** These contracts are built around a tier system that groups procedural codes into specific tiers and assigns payment obligation to each tier. The procedures within each tier are normally of similar complexity and require a similar level of time, skill, and expertise. Each payer has its own tier system, although the more complex procedures earn higher reimbursement from the majority of commercial payers.

## Knowing the rules governing which codes you can use

When you're coding, you just look at the fee schedule, find the CPT codes you need, and include them all on the claim form, right? Wrong. Not every code can be grouped or classified similarly, so you have to know what kind of code you're dealing with:

✔ **Codes that can't be billed with other codes:** Codes that represent different procedures to the same body part often can't be billed together. For example, an open reduction (or repair through an incision) of a fracture of the radius can't be billed with a closed reduction (setting the fracture without an incision) of the same body part. In these cases, only the more complex procedure is billed. When would such a situation occur? Suppose the physician tries a less invasive procedure but is unable to attain the desired results, so she ends up performing a more invasive or complex procedure. Only the more invasive or complex procedure is billable.

To understand what can and can't be billed separately, you need to understand bundling. The later section "Paying attention to your bundle of joy" has the details.

✔ **Codes for procedures that can't be billed under specific circumstances:** Men can't get hysterectomies, so if a claim for a male patient lists a code for a hysterectomy, the payer isn't going to pay the claim. For obvious reasons, a hysterectomy is a procedure that is only payable if the patient is female.

✔ **Codes that can only be billed to a patient once in a life time:** We only have one of some things (like gallbladders, spleens, and uteruses); therefore, a patient can have such an organ removed only once. If the payer system is up to date, additional claims for these types of one-time-only procedures are always rejected.

✔ **Codes that require specific conditions to be met before they can be billed:** Some codes are age related, others are sex related, and still others are the one-time only codes (explained in the preceding item in the list). For example, various procedures (such as tonsillectomies or adenoid removals) are appropriate only for specific age groups. The CPT book indicates when a procedure code has such a condition.

✔ **Codes that aren't compatible with other codes (at least in theory):** Sometimes codes just can't be combined because performing both procedures would 1) be impossible, 2) not make sense, or 3) represent a service or procedure that is incidental to another. For example, you wouldn't submit a procedure code for a right foot bunion repair during the same session when the right foot was amputated. Why would a physician bother with the bunion if the foot's coming off anyway? Well, he wouldn't, which is why you simply can't combine those codes. The same holds true with a cataract extraction for an eye that was removed the previous month, or an appendectomy performed on a patient during the same session as a colectomy (colon removal). These codes can't be combined because the procedures can't be done at the same time.

You can find out more about these unlikely — and often a bit humorous — coding scenarios by checking out Medicare's set of edits known as Medically Unlikely Edits (MUEs). These edits are available on the Centers for Medicare & Medicaid Services (CMS) website (www.cms.gov) and on most Medicare contractor websites.

---

## Revenue codes

Revenue codes are four-digit codes that are used on UB-04 claim forms, the forms used by facilities to bill most commercial payers. Revenue codes are only used on UB-04 claim forms; they're also used in addition to CPT codes. They let the payer know what kind of procedures the submitting provider is contracted or licensed to perform and bill. For providers, such as a hospital with multiple locations, the revenue code identifies the department in which the procedure was performed.

Providers that submit revenue codes have the accepted revenue codes specified in each vendor contract. The specific revenue codes listed in the contracts are discussed on the AAPC website (www.aapc.com) and are also discussed in the Medicare Internet Only Processing manual, which you can access on the CMS website: www.cms.gov.

Although facility claims are submitted on UB-04 claim forms, professional claims are submitted on HCFA/CMS-1500 claim forms, which represent the services performed by a physician or other professional healthcare provider.

I discuss the differences in the forms in Chapter 2. What's important to remember here is that, although revenue codes only show up on the UB-04 form, they are somewhat related to what can be found on the HCFA/CMS-1500, and both kinds of forms must be as accurate as possible.

---

## Linking your CPT codes to ICD-9 codes

Remember your good friend, medical necessity (if you don't, refer to Chapter 5)? Medical necessity plays a big role when it comes to the viability of the procedure codes you use. Every CPT code billed must be supported by a corresponding ICD-9 diagnosis code that supports medical necessity for the procedure that was performed.

One diagnosis may support several procedure codes. A patient who presents with ankle instability may require as many as three billable procedures to stabilize the joint, and all three of these procedures will be paid. All of this information is part of the medical record; you just need to play Sherlock Holmes to find the coding clues to identify any and all billable codes.

## Making your code as specific as possible

In addition to choosing the right code, you also need to ensure that the assigned code is specific to the procedure. Just as you rely on the physician to be as specific as possible in his or her documentation, the physician relies on you to assign the most accurate codes possible.

For this process to work as it should, two things need to happen, in the following order: First, the physician needs to document correctly so that you can choose the appropriate procedural code. Second, you use the physician's documentation to choose the correct CPT code. The next sections have the details.

### The doc's job: Documenting diagnosis and procedure

In the physician documentation, the physician must clearly state and describe the procedure that was performed. Here's an example of good documentation; it has everything you need to select the correct codes:

> A longitudinal incision was made to the radial aspect of the DIP joint of the left index finger. Subcutaneous dissection was blunt. An obvious ganglion was identified. The connection to the joint between the extensor tendon and collateral ligament was identified. The joint was opened, and the cyst was removed in its entirety, leaving the ligaments intact. The wound was irrigated. A vicryl stitch was placed between the tendon and the ligament. The skin was closed, and a dressing was applied.

Seems simple enough, right? Unfortunately, you'll occasionally encounter the following problems, which need to be resolved before you can assign the proper codes:

✔ **A physician simply dictates that he performed a specific procedure, but instead of describing the procedure, he uses a CPT code.** For example, "I then performed a CPT 29828." This type of entry doesn't satisfy documentation requirements. The physician must describe the procedure in detail before it you can code and bill it. Proper documentation of a surgical procedure includes a brief history of the patient's problem, a good dictation of the approach taken, any structures affected by the approach, a clear description of what was done while inside the patient, any complications that may have arisen, and an explanation of the closure and recovery.

✔ **A physician may consistently fail to document a particular procedure, saying, "That's what I always mean when I say that."** Unfortunately, his intentions don't constitute proper documentation. The physician must clearly state and describe the procedure that was performed each and every time he performs it.

If you're dealing with a doc who habitually makes these documentation assumptions, you may have to produce the necessary documentation— that is, show him the description of the procedure as published by the AMA or CMS — so that he agrees to comply. Doing so is more work for you, but it pays off big time later when you file that clean claim.

In these situations, you need to get the missing information; after all, it's the physician's job to describe procedures, and it's your job to code them, not the other way around. However, how you go about filling in the documentation blanks is very important. You can't ask leading questions, for example, because doing so can lead to fraudulent coding and excessive reimbursement. Head to the later section "Setting the record straight: Physician queries" for strategies you can use to get the info you need.

### The coder's job: Choosing the correct CPT codes

Most of the procedural codes are well-defined by the American Medical Association. They describe specifically how physicians have been trained to perform the procedures. For example, CPT 25609 is the open reduction with internal fixation of an intra-articular (in the joint) distal radius fracture. (In plain English, this is a surgical procedure in which a broken arm is repaired through an incision). This description reflects the industry standard regarding how the procedure is performed.

Every CPT code has a specific description. The documentation should fully support the use of each CPT code you submit for payment. In this game, close isn't good enough. The code has to be exact; you can't choose a code that's merely similar. Occasionally, however, you may have to use an *unspecified code* (which is pretty much what it sounds like — a code that is used when no other specific code fits).

Unspecified codes exist because the CPT codes aren't set in stone. As technology evolves, so do procedural codes. When a new technique is developed or modified as a result of new technology, the previously used code may no longer be appropriate. With an unspecified code, you compare the pricing to a similar specified code. For example, arthroscopic biceps tenotomy (cutting the tendon) currently doesn't have a specific CPT code, so when that procedure is performed, coders use CPT 29999 and compare it for pricing purposes to CPT 23405, which is the code that would be used if the procedure had been done through a traditional incision.

## Paying attention to your bundle of joy

You can link some services together when you code because a physician may have performed one service as the result of doing another. As luck would have it, there's a handy-dandy term for grouping services under one code: *bundling*. Other times, codes describing services considered to be inclusive to each other (that is, performed as part of a single procedure) can be billed separately.

Knowing what to bundle or not is a skill that comes with practice and learning the ins and outs of your coding resource books. Refer to Chapter 4 for detailed info on bundling. In the next sections, I give you a quick overview.

### Bundling basics

Whether procedures can be billed separately or not depends on what goes on during the surgery:

✔ If additional skill and time are required to do the extra work, then the other procedure may qualify for additional reimbursement. For example, closure of a surgical opening is part of the surgery. But if the closure is a complex procedure that involves an extensive amount of time and skill, then you may be able to *unbundle* those services. Unbundling means that two or more codes that are normally incidental to another can be billed separately. To do that, you apply the individual codes and a modifier to bypass the edit.

✔ If the physician performed the procedure because he was already working on that part of the body, it's incidental and *not* separately billable. If, for example, a surgeon is performing abdominal surgery and decides to remove the patient's appendix as well, you can't bill for the appendectomy, because the surgeon was already in there.

✔ Bundling can refer to a procedure that had to be done to successfully complete the primary procedure. Think about incisions and repairs. Before a surgeon can enter the body, an incision has to be made; therefore, it's not really a separate procedure. After the physician completes the surgery, the incision needs to be closed. Closure is not separate; it's a pretty important part of the procedure.

If you use coding software, the software indicates when two or more procedures are incidental to another. If you don't use coding software, you can go to the Medicare website and most Medicare contractor websites to find out what the proper edit is.

You use *modifiers* to indicate that the procedure being billed has been modified or altered from its published description. You don't use them purely to seek additional reimbursement. To find out more about modifiers, head to the later section "Using Modifiers Correctly."

### Dealing with bundling errors

Most payer processing software programs identify bundling errors, or more accurately, they identify procedures that have been unbundled improperly. They don't identify procedures that *should* have been included but that are missing. (After all, payers don't want to pay more than they must. If you unbundle for additional reimbursement, and the payer doesn't agree that the extra reimbursement is supported, it won't pay for it.) It's your responsibility as the coder to review the medical documentation and identify all billable procedural codes.

Not all payer processing software identifies bundling errors. If you submit claims to those payers, the claim will pay as you billed it. Keep in mind, however, that this doesn't give you carte blanche to over-code. When you *over-code,* you take advantage of payers by submitting procedures that will pay but that are not supported in the record. The provider you work for is bound by ethics to submit truthful claims. Just because a payer will allow it, doesn't mean you should bill it when unbundling is not supported.

# Using Modifiers Correctly

You use modifiers to alter the description of a service or supply that has been provided. You can use modifiers in circumstances such as the following:

✔ **The service or procedure has both a professional and technical component.** An example would be radiological procedures: One provider (the facility) owns the equipment and bears the cost of maintenance and other things, but the physician must interpret the findings of the radiological procedure.

✔ **The service or procedure was performed by more than one physician and/or in more than one location.** For a complex procedure that requires more than two hands, an assistant surgeon may be used.

✔ **The service or procedure has been increased or reduced.** For example, a procedure that normally takes an hour requires two hours because of scar tissue, or the description of a procedure notes that another procedure is included but that other procedure wasn't necessary and therefore wasn't performed.

✔ **Only part of a service was performed.** A procedure that is bilateral by definition (that is, it is performed on both sides) is performed only on one side.

✔ **The service or procedure was provided more than once.** An example would be excising lesions on different areas of one body part through separate incisions.

✔ **Events occurred that were unusual to the circumstances.** For example, the patient had an adverse reaction to anesthesia which resulted in early termination.

Payer organizations revise modifiers annually, with some being added and others deleted, and each payer can determine whether and how the modifiers must be used for its own organization. For example, Medicare discontinued the SG modifier, which it once used to indicate that a claim was for a facility, but various Medicaid and Workers' Compensation payers still require it. For this reason, you must keep abreast of individual payer preferences with regard to required modifiers.

While some payers require modifiers, others don't care whether modifiers are applied because their contracts pay based on the revenue codes or the procedure codes. Using a modifier for these claims usually doesn't affect payment. What affects payment is failing to apply modifiers that are required by the individual payers.

Because commercial payer policies differ, make sure you have access to their contracts so that you can code the claims correctly with the required modifiers. You're also responsible for remaining current with regard to modifiers your employer uses. You can find modifiers in the CPT book, on the CMS website (www.cms.gov), and on Medicare contractor websites.

In the following sections, you can read about how modifiers relate to commercial payers as well as government ones. Other government payers such as the Department of Labor, Medicaid and TRICOR have specific modifier requirements for various classifications of providers and procedures.

## *Using modifiers for commercial payers*

To apply more specific payments to procedures, many commercial payers require modifiers. Keep in mind, though, that how the modifiers are used differs from payer to payer. The following sections show some examples.

### *Modifiers 50, 52, RT, and LT*

Certain procedural codes are bilateral in their description (that is, the procedure is performed on both sides of the body), while others require the use of a modifier to indicate laterality. Modifier 50 indicates that a procedure was performed bilaterally. If a provider performs a bilateral procedure on one side only, the coder must apply modifier 52 to indicate that the services were reduced.

Some commercial payers recognize the 50 modifiers, essentially agreeing that the procedure was performed twice, once on each side — and process accordingly. Other providers require that the procedure be listed twice on the claim, first with the modifier LT (meaning "left") and then again with the modifier RT (right).

### *TC modifier and modifiers 22 and 26*

Commercial payers commonly use the TC modifier and Modifier 22:

- ✔ **TC modifier and modifier 26:** TC means "technical component." When a radiology service is being billed, for example, the facility that owns the equipment can bill for its use by applying the TC modifier to the appropriate procedural code. The physician who interprets the X-ray or other product of the radiology service can report his services by billing the same procedural code with a 26 modifier, indicating that the physician who didn't own the equipment did this work.

✔ **Modifier 22:** This modifier is used when a procedure is more extensive or required more time and skill than normal.

## Using modifiers for Medicare

Medicare claims always require the use of appropriate modifiers such as the following:

✔ Modifiers that indicate laterality.

✔ Modifiers that indicate services were provided by resident medical students. It may also require a specific modifier to indicate that the reason another physician assisted was because a resident physician was unavailable. (*Resident physicians* are no longer medical students but are still in the learning phase of their careers. They have MD behind their names but continue to work with supervision before taking board examinations.)

✔ Modifiers to indicate that a non-physician practitioner, such as a nurse practitioner or a physician assistant, provided a service. Another modifier indicates that a non-physician who assisted a physician is seeking a separate reimbursement (applicable only if the procedural code is one that has been determined to require the additional assistance).

For additional information about Medicare modifier requirements, go to the CMS website (www.cms.gov).

## Using modifiers for other government payers

In addition to Medicare, other government payers require modifiers, as the next sections explain.

### Tricare

Tricare, funded by the Department of Defense, insures active military members and their eligible dependents, as well as retired military members who have chosen to exercise the option to remain covered and their dependents. The options available to patients depend on their military status and where they live.

Tricare's processing software accepts all current modifiers, so when you bill this carrier, you want to make sure that you use all applicable modifiers. For example, a patient may have surgery for a hernia, which has a 90 day global package. (Tricare *global packages* specify the number of days and the services — preoperative assessment, postoperative visits, and so on — included with the reimbursement for the procedure.) That same patient may later see the same physician for a different ailment that requires a separate and appropriate modifier in order to be paid.

Tricare benefits are administered through three Tricare area administrators: Tricare North, Tricare South, and Tricare West. Each of these administrators maintains a website that allows providers to verify fee schedules, check on required modifiers, and view other payer specific information.

### Workers' Comp (The Department of Labor)

The Department of Labor recognizes current modifiers as determined by Medicare, but they still determine payment based on the approved procedure and diagnosis codes regardless of the modifiers.

## Using retired modifiers

Certain payers use older claims processing systems. Many of the Medicaid payers and some of the smaller Workers' Compensation payers still use these older programs and, as a result, still require the use of retired modifiers. *Retired modifiers* are those that were removed from the Medicare list.

One retired modifier that is still routinely used is the SG modifier, mentioned earlier. This modifier was used to indicate that the procedure code on the claim was being submitted by an ambulatory surgery center (ASC) to represent that share of the service provided.

You're responsible for knowing which modifiers the payer requires. If you submit a claim without the appropriate modifier or with a new modifier that isn't programmed into the payer's processing software, the claim will reject. To prevent this from happening and to get the claim paid faster, always check with the payer prior to submission. If the payer is one of those who doesn't answer the phone or hasn't updated its website with current policies, you need to follow up with a letter. In the letter, request a summary of claim filing requirements.

## Checking for Money Left on the Table

Your responsibility as a biller/coder is to abstract all billable codes from the medical record. Failing to identify billable codes (*under-coding*) is referred to as leaving money on the table. And leaving money on the table will get you fired. Want to understand and avoid under-coding? Read on.

As bad as under-coding is, over-coding is just as bad. When payers discover later that a claim was over paid, they'll ask for the money back, usually in the form of a demand letter that describes the over payment and explains why the payment should be returned. If the payment isn't returned, the payer uses the over-payment as an offset to future claims, sort of like a credit, in what is known as a *take-back*. Take-backs are a challenge to the payer, but they're even more of a challenge for the provider because convincing a payer that the overpayment doesn't actually exist can be difficult. When the payer has already used the perceived overpayment toward future claims, the ledger can get pretty messy.

Some states have laws that define the number of months that can pass in which an overpayment refund can be requested. These state laws don't apply to federal plans. Some state laws also define the time frame in which carriers can request payment returns. Make sure you know the laws of your state.

## Turning a critical eye to the record

You must catch any and every service in the provider's record and code it accordingly. Unfortunately, although the coding software your provider uses may help you identify a lot of oddities in the claim, such as unbundling, it won't help you identify under-coding. To do that, you have to rely on your coding skills, because you're the last line of defense against leaving money on the table.

If your employer doesn't use coding software, the National Correct Coding edits are available on the Medicare website as well as most of the Medicare contractor websites. Other sources include coding companion publications that usually indicate procedures that are inclusive to a particular code.

Under-coding errors often result from a misunderstanding about what can and can't be bundled. Although you don't want to over-code, you do want to look critically at every procedure so that you can determine whether you can code it separately.

## Overriding published edits

As the coder, you can override — or bypass — a published edit in the software, if you know how. The most obvious way to bypass a published edit is to assign a modifier to a code. This modifier gives the payer more information about the procedure in question. As I explain earlier, modifiers indicate when a procedure has been altered from its published description and should be reimbursed accordingly. They may indicate that a normally bundled procedure was actually separate or that a procedure required additional time and work by the physician or required assistance of a co-surgeon or assistant surgeon among other things.

In some circumstances, you can't use a modifier, even though, when reviewing the record, you can clearly see that the provider performed extra work. In this situation, if you're dealing with a commercial payer, you may be able to convince the payer to allow the additional procedures. Keep in mind, though, that if these payers base their argument on edits found in their own claim editing software and the edit says "no," then the answer is "no."

Payers use different claim-editing programs that may differ from the NCCI edits and can be frustrating to providers. Usually the payer contracts identify which claims editing software they use for processing. Some payers use more than one type of editing software and apply the one that allows them to pay the least. Again, this situation is frustrating for providers, and if it's in the contract, it can be very hard to challenge successfully.

## Setting the record straight: Physician queries

So you've coded the claim and see that you still have money on the table, or procedures that were under-coded. Time to go back to the source — the doc. Why? Because if poor documentation is the cause of money being left on the table, then you need to communicate with the physician to find out what may be missing in the record.

### Knowing when a physician query is necessary

When you ask for clarification, you're performing what is known as a *physician query*. A physician query is necessary when you encounter an implied procedure or a missing procedure:

- ✓ **Implied procedure:** In this situation, a procedure may be listed in the heading of a record, but it's not documented in the body of the record.

- ✓ **Missing procedure:** A missing procedure is one for which a diagnosis is listed but no treatment is noted.

The missing or implied procedure may have been a result of the physician being interrupted during dictation, or it may be an error in transcription. Most physicians and facilities use transcription services. The physician dictates, and the transcriptionist listens to the dictation and types the words into a document. Sometimes the transcriptionist uses templates and fails to import the correct one. Other providers use voice recognition software. The physician dictates, and the words are entered automatically into a document. These notes have frequent errors, and clarification of the medical record is important for legal reasons.

If you work with a particular physician for an extended time, you'll be so familiar with what the doctor does and how he does it that you'll essentially be "in the doctor's head" every time you read the documentation. It's vitally important that you remain cognizant of the need for clear documentation and are careful about not coding a procedure that likely was done but is omitted from the documentation.

### Conducting a physician query

A physician query is simply a note to the physician that asks for clarification of the record. Some offices have a query form you can use to seek clarification when a procedure has been implied or is obviously missing. Many of these forms, which are common in hospitals or large offices, list the most common omissions and a line for "Other." You simply check the box you need more information for.

If you work for different providers, you need to familiarize yourself with the various query procedures of each office. If you're working with a small office or practice, you can leave the note or chart in question on the physician's desk with a note that says something like: "Which arm was it?" or "How large was the lesion?"

In other practices, you can simply ask the physician a non-leading question, and the provider will then dictate an addendum to the record that clarifies or corrects the issue at hand. Knowing how to approach the physicians now can help you produce sparkly clean claims later.

When you ask a physician for clarification about a record, beware of putting words in the doc's mouth. Any and all clarification about records must come straight from the physician — not you. Don't make assumptions about what he meant. Question the documentation, but don't lead. Here are some examples of good versus bad queries:

| *Instead of This* | *Say This* |
| --- | --- |
| It was the left arm, correct? | What arm did you perform the procedure on? |
| Was the tumor more than 5 cm? | How large was the tumor? |
| Did you excise more than 1 cm of clavicle? | How much clavicle was removed? |
| Did you debride to bleeding bone? | How extensive was the debridement? |

# Checking and Double-Checking Your Documentation

Just as carpenters "measure twice, cut once," before you send out a claim, you need to check and double check your work to increase your chances for success (read, getting the requested reimbursement) the first time around.

Submitting a claim correctly with all necessary information required for prompt processing is known as filing a "clean" claim. A clean claim is one that can be processed without the payer needing to request additional information from the provider or a third party.

When you review each record during your final check for accuracy, remember to do the following:

- ✔ Make sure that the patient name, address, date of birth, identification number, and group number are correct and populate the correct fields.

- ✔ Check to see that all billable codes are documented.

- ✔ Verify that the form contains no expired or deleted codes and that the codes have been entered correctly (no transposed digits).

- ✔ Verify that medical necessity has been met.

  You must make sure that the documentation is relative to the diagnosis. The record should always include the reason for the patient encounter (medical necessity, which you can read more about in Chapter 5). In addition, any and all procedural codes submitted for payment must be supported by the appropriate diagnosis code that supports medical necessity. When a diagnosis is entered into the record, a decision regarding treatment usually follows it, if it wasn't actually treated at that time. Diagnosis codes such as these that are part of the medical record but that seem to just "be there" may also be subject to physician query. If a billable procedure is obviously missing, indicate that to the physician. Ask her to clarify the record. Refer to the earlier section "Setting the record straight: Physician Queries" for details.

- ✔ Make sure the record is complete and that all fields are populated.

- ✔ Check that all required signatures are dated, especially physician signatures. Electronic signatures also show a time and date stamp.

- ✔ If the physician completed a super-bill (a billing form used in many providers offices that includes the most frequently performed procedures), verify that the procedures indicated on the bill are documented in the record.

- ✔ Verify the prioritization of the codes in relation to the payer-specific contract. Know which codes are obligated for higher reimbursement. (The payer may want the highest paying code listed first on the claim.)

> ✔ Check for bundling/unbundling issues. You can find out more about these in the earlier section "Paying attention to your bundle of joy."
>
> ✔ Make sure that the payer is correctly identified, including the right payer identification number and payer mailing address.

After you make sure that all of these elements are in place, you submit that puppy! The preferred method of submitting claims is electronically. Electronic submission is faster, and it allows the provider to verify that the payer accepted the claim. The clearinghouse will acknowledge the receipt of each claim and will also generate an acceptance report if one is returned by the payer after the assigned payer has accepted the claim. For more information on what happens in the clearinghouse and beyond, head to Chapter 13.

## Keeping paper claims clean

Although paper claims can be a nightmare to keep clean, they are necessary at times. When you have to submit a claim on paper, follow these guidelines:

✔ Use only original claim forms (the ones printed in red). The current acceptable forms are the CMS-1500 and the UB-04. (Make sure you're using the correct edition of the form. On the CMS-1500 form, look for "Approved by National Uniform Claim Committee [with the most recent date of approval]" at the top of the form, and "Approved OMB-xxxx-xxxx Form CMS -1500 [date]" in the bottom right-hand corner.)

✔ If you need to write on the claim for any reason, use blue or black ink. The payer processing software does not recognize red ink because the forms are red. (Also keep in mind that some payers don't accept claims with anything written on them by hand.)

✔ Do not submit totally handwritten claims.

✔ Make sure that the print on the claims is dark.

✔ If the toner in your printer is starting to run low, it may leave blank streaks. Do not send claims out with these streaks.

✔ Claims scan best when you use at least a size 12 font in uppercase letters. Make sure that the information that is required in each field prints within the area of each block.

✔ Processing software doesn't recognize punctuation, so don't use it. Nor do you need to use decimal points (separate fields exist for dollars and cents).

✔ Don't send attachments unless the payer requires them.

Paper claims are difficult to track and take longer to reach the payer. If you are forced to submit multiple paper claims to an individual payer, send them certified or registered mail so that you have proof that the claims reached the payer and that somebody at that office accepted the package. Also check on these claims within a week to make sure that they have been entered into the payer processing system. When you call to follow up a paper claim, let the representative know that the claim was submitted on paper and the date it was sent.

Remember that insurance companies are in business to make money for their investors, and they'll use any excuse to reject your claim. Paper claims require more handling by the payer, which increases the chances of the claim being entered incorrectly or even lost.

# Chapter 13

# From Clearinghouse to Accounts Receivable to Money in the Pocket

---

## In This Chapter

▶ Linking RVUs and prioritization to reimbursement amounts

▶ Decreasing the time your claims linger in accounts receivable

▶ Using explanation of benefits documentation to verify proper payment

---

$A$s the preceding chapters make clear, a lot goes into getting a claim ready, and nearly an entire village has had its fingers in the pie. The front office staff has gathered all of the necessary demographic and insurance information. The physician has seen the patient and documented all provided services in the medical record. You have carefully abstracted all billable services and supported them with diagnosis codes that support medical necessity, entered the insurance and demographics information and the codes into the billing software, reviewed everything to make sure all the *i*'s are dotted and *t*'s crossed, and then sent the claim on its way with a kiss, a wave, and silent prayer that it doesn't take to drinking or get caught up with the wrong crowd.

Yes, a lot can happen to a claim once it leaves your conscientious hands. In this chapter, you take a look at the kinds of things — beyond coding errors — that can impact whether your claim generates the payments your provider deserves. I also explain some of the things that impact the final reimbursement amount.

## Spending Time in the Clearinghouse

When the claim is ready to be submitted, you upload it to the clearinghouse to be sent to the payer. What, exactly, happens once your claim reaches the clearinghouse? The next sections explain.

## Scrub-a-dub-dub: Checking for errors

At the clearinghouse the claim is *scrubbed*, or checked for errors. Some errors identified by the clearinghouse can be corrected online so that the claim can be forwarded on. This type of error includes mistakes regarding revenue codes or other clerical issues. Other errors, however, are not so easily fixable. For these, the claim needs to be fixed at the provider's office and then resubmitted. Errors of this type include attempting to submit to a payer who is unknown to the clearinghouse. This situation can occur because some smaller payers don't accept electronic claims and aren't registered with any of the clearinghouse companies. In this case, you must submit a paper claim directly to the payer. (Directions for claim submission are always noted on the patient's ID card.)

## Matchmaker, matchmaker: Sending the claim to the right payer

The clearinghouse directs the claim to the payer, according to the payer identification number, in a process known as *payer matching*. During the provider's original enrollment with the clearinghouse, payers are matched to the correct payer identification number following the first claim submission. The payer ID is the electronic address of the payer, and it tells the clearinghouse where to send the claim. Every time a claim is submitted to a new payer, the clearinghouse flags the claim for payer matching.

The provider is responsible for telling the clearinghouse which payer should receive the claim. If the provider identifies the wrong payer, the claim won't be paid. (Payers don't take claims that belong to other insurance companies and send them on. Instead, the payer usually rejects the claim and sends notice of that rejection to the submitting provider.)

The payer processes the claim and determines the reimbursement according to the codes submitted on the claim. For info on what goes on after the claim is in the payer's hands, head to the later section "Payment or Denial: Being in the Hands of the Payer."

Revenue codes are not usually assigned by the coder, but they are programmed into the billing software and are based on the type of provider submitting the claim.

## Generating reports

Every clearinghouse keeps track of the claims that pass through its system. Reports are available that show claims that were sent, which payer they were sent to, and when all of these transactions occurred. Also available are reports that indicate when a problem occurs with claim submission. You can find these reports on the provider's clearinghouse web page. Most payers also send files back to the clearinghouse that report the status of the transmitted file(s).

Sometimes a provider submits an incorrect claim, isn't notified of an error, and the claim just seems to disappear. This is why follow up is so important. Be sure to check the clearinghouse acceptance reports and verify them with the billing software submitted claims, also called the *batch report,* daily. If a claim is on the batch report but not on the acceptance report, find out why.

Daily verification of the rejected reports is also important. Part of your office routine should be to check the rejection report and fix all claims on the same day if possible. By following up immediately, you can prevent timely filing denials (that is, having your claim denied because you failed to submit it within the payer's published timeframe).

# Factors Affecting Reimbursement Amounts

Claims are submitted to generate reimbursement. Each provider determines how much it will charge for services provided, but that is not necessarily the fee that the payers will pay. When a provider and payer have a contract, reimbursement is based entirely on the obligation that is contractually defined. Without a contract, reimbursement depends on different factors, which I discuss in the following sections.

## Understanding relative value units

You may wonder how CPT codes correspond to a dollar value and why. The system used by Medicare and many HMOs is called the Resource Based Relative Value Scale (RBRVS). Every CPT code has been assigned something called a relative value unit, or RVU, that determines the cost of a service.

### Determining the RVU

The RVU is determined by first adding up three components:

- **The work required by the physician:** This component takes into consideration the amount of time, skill, training, and intensity that was necessary to perform the procedure. Each CPT code is reviewed at least every five years to determine whether this value should remain the same.

- **The cost of doing business or maintaining a practice:** This includes rent, equipment, supplies, and staff.

✔ **The malpractice expense or liability expenses borne by the provider:** Malpractice/liability expenses vary among providers. Certain specialties such as obstetrics tend to involve higher malpractice premiums than a primary care physician is likely to face.

These three RVU factors are then multiplied by a geographical adjustment that creates the compensation level for the service in that exact location. (This geographical adjustment explains why a procedure done in New York City is worth more than the same procedure done in Boise.) The geographically adjusted RVUs are then multiplied by a conversion factor that converts the RVU into a dollar amount, which determines the price that Medicare or the HMO pays. Using this formula, any entity can calculate the price it'll reimburse for any given procedure.

### RVUs and contract details

Make sure that you know the contract details for each payer, because the differences between payers can be huge. For example, depending upon how the contract is structured, the providers may still find themselves paid per RVU rather than contract allowance.

Also, when multiple procedures are billed on a claim, they are prioritized for payment, and a discount, called the *multiple procedure discount* (*MPD*), is often applied. The procedure that is obligated at the higher allowance is paid at 100 percent of the allowed amount; the second procedure may be paid at 50 percent; and so on. On contracts that are based on RVUs, the higher the RVU, the higher priority for payment. You can read more about prioritization of payments in the next section.

Not all contracts are RVU-based, and procedures that are obligated to pay higher according to the contract may have a lower RVU. This sometimes occurs when the contract contains several commonly performed procedures that have been carved out. With this tactic (which is referred to as *strategic contract management*), specialty providers identify certain procedures that are routinely performed and ask that one or two (or more) of the related procedural codes be *carved out*, or especially identified as payable at a flat rate that isn't linked to RVUs or any other fee schedule. A surgeon who performs 300 laparoscopic cholecystectomies (gallbladder removals) each year may try to have that specific procedural code carved out of one or two of his network contracts to pay a flat rate.

## Prioritization of procedures

The payment poster, the person who posts the payments to the account ledger, needs to know the correct order in which to post the payment. He gets that info from the claim form.

Procedures are billed by order of expected payment. The procedure that is expected to reimburse the greatest amount needs to be the first one listed on the claim, the procedure that is expected to reimburse the next greatest amount is next on the claim form, and so on down the line.

How this order is established varies. Many offices have the contract pricing programmed into their billing software. If the software is programmed correctly (that is, the contracts are loaded correctly, and the claim is linked to the correct payer contract in the billing software), the claim will be submitted in the correct order. (*Note:* The program should be updated every year and every time the contract is revised.)

If the software is not programmed, then the responsibility for prioritization of procedures falls to you. That is why you need to know the contractual obligation for each procedure — so that you can identify which procedure is to pay at 100 percent and so on.

Most payers have processing software that recognizes the correct prioritization of the procedures and processes the claim to pay in that order, but some payers pay claims based solely on the prioritization established by the billing provider. That's why it's important to know whether the payer is contracted. If so, the highest reimbursable procedure will likely be listed first on the claim, followed by the next higher, and so on. But if the payer contract is RVU-based rather than procedural based, the procedure with the highest RVU is first.

If an error occurs in claims payment, the problem may be the prioritization. If the provider thinks a certain CPT code should have paid at 100 percent of allowed, but that CPT has a lower RVU and the payer software processes per RVU, a dispute is certain. In such cases, the contract prevails, so you need to know the contract and your priorities — literally! In the end, the payer is the one who decides whether to make payment. Most contracts contain arbitration clauses that outline the process of dispute resolution. When no contract is in place, the dispute can escalate to a legal issue to be decided by a judge.

# Payment or Denial: Being in the Hands of the Payer

After you submit the claim to the clearinghouse and the clearinghouse acknowledges the receipt of the claim and sends it off to the payer, you wait. Every payer has its own timetable and, depending on how clean your claim is (refer to Chapter 12), will choose to push things through the system or deny your claim.

Diligent claim follow up on your part can accelerate prompt payment. This process needs to begin the day that the claim is uploaded to the clearinghouse. Be sure to verify and archive all transmission reports. These reports are your proof that the claim was sent, and they serve as proof of timely filing should a dispute occur later.

After accepting the claim (either in electronic or paper form), the payer either rejects it or sends it for processing. When the payer enters the claim for processing, it is referred to as a *pending claim,* which means it's waiting to be reviewed for payment. Fortunately, you can do things to shorten the wait time, which I explain in the next section.

After that, the claim will either be paid or. . . not. If your provider gets paid, you're golden. If not, you have to deal with rejection or the big D — denial. The following sections have the details.

## *Reducing your time in accounts receivable*

The practice of following up claims after submission can reduce the number of days from submission date to payment date. Ideally, the claim should leave your hands within 72 hours after the date of service. That is when the payment clock starts and when you can start looking for that check to show up in accounts receivable (AR).

To help reduce your claim's time in AR, state payment laws legislate the number of days in which a payer must pay a clean claim. Payer contacts usually have prompt pay clauses, as well.

Your billing software can help you keep track of how long a claim has gone unpaid by giving providers access to a number of reports. One of those is the *aged collection ledger.* This report reflects the individual payers and the patient accounts that are associated with each payer. The report also indicates the age of the account in number of days; 30 days or less, 31–60 days, 61–90 days, 91–120 days, and so on. The report also shows the number of days allowed in AR per payer.

When looking at the report, look at the abbreviated version, which is the age of the accounts per payer, and do the following:

1. **Beginning with the payer with the largest number of accounts receivable outstanding, look at the payer's accounts that are 30 days or less.**

   Verify that these claims have been received. Doing so helps prevent timely filing issues later on.

2. **Looking at the oldest accounts, call each payer and check the status of each account.**

   Here are some questions to ask each payer you call:

   - "Has a claim number been assigned? If so, what is it?"
   - "What is the status of this claim?"
   - "When can we expect payment?"
   - "Are there any issues causing the claim to be delayed? If so, how can we fix them?"
   - "Is additional information needed?" If so, get a fax number and send the necessary information; then call back and confirm the receipt of the fax.
   - "With whom am I speaking, and what is the reference number for this call?"

3. **Work your way through the aged account ledger by looking at the accounts as they have aged and get the claims in process to pay.**

   If you are responsible for the financial state of the aged accounts, the fewer the days in accounts receivable for each claim, the better you look.

## Overcoming rejection

With a rejection, essential information is missing from the claim that prevents the payer from entering the claim into its system. Common reasons for rejection include missing or incorrect patient identification number or demographic information such as sex or birth date. Your goal with a rejection is to provide the missing info in a thorough and timely manner.

If a claim doesn't process correctly as result of a coding error, you need to submit a corrected claim. Many payers have specific forms that you must use to facilitate this process. Usually the form asks for the original claim number and includes a field you use to identify the reason for the corrected claim submission.

 If you notice that a claim was coded or billed incorrectly, it's the provider's responsibility to notify the payer of the error. Failing to notify a payer when a claim has been erroneously submitted may result in charges of fraud. Other types of fraud include knowingly submitting incorrect information or filing a claim for services that were not provided.

In some cases, the payer may request a refund of the incorrectly billed claim. Medicare has a voluntary refund form on the Centers for Medicare & Medicaid Services (CMS) website, as do most carrier websites. This form is used when a provider wants to return a Medicare payment, and it allows the provider to simply submit a new claim. Commercial payers vary in their policies when dealing with an incorrectly submitted claim, so check with the individual payer to verify the process prior to sending back a payment.

## Dealing with denial

Reimbursement is a direct result of the provider's tenacity in following up the claim submission and submitting claims correctly. Claim errors result in either rejections (covered in the preceding section) or denials. With a denial, the claim went through the provider but is not being paid for some reason. Claims deny for a myriad of reasons, such as omission of policyholder information (name, birthdate, and relationship to patient) when different than the patient, failure to obtain an authorization number or referral, not checking the "Accept Assignment" box, or missing or incomplete provider information, such as the physical address where services were rendered.

When you're faced with a denial, you don't take it lying down. Instead, you gather together your wherewithal, your documentation, and anything else you need and file an appeal. The next chapter has the details.

# Breaking Down the EOB

After a claim processes, payment follows. Each payment is accompanied by an *explanation of benefits*, or EOB. The EOB is sent to the patient and the provider to show how the claim processed. It also lets the provider know whether any remaining balance is due by the patient. As a biller/coder, you want to review this documentation to verify that the claim has processed and paid correctly.

## Getting familiar with an EOB

An EOB generally contains the details explaining how the claim was processed, although some payer EOBs show only the total claim amount, along with the total provider write off, and the total allowance. When this happens, it is up to the payment poster, or designee, to break the payment out to show the detail by line.

On the EOB, payments are posted by line item. If a claim has four CPT codes on it, then the payment is allocated among the payable four lines to show how much reimbursement was received for each procedure.

Here are the kinds of postings you see on the EOB for every CPT code listed:

- ✔ Amount of the procedure before any discounts are applied

- ✔ Amount that the patient is responsible for

- ✔ How much the contract allows for the procedure

- ✔ The type and amount of any discounts that apply

- ✔ The final amount of the reimbursement after all discounts, deductibles, and so on are applied

As a coder, you need to pay attention to the details on this form to make sure the provider received the reimbursement to which she was entitled. Here are some things to look for:

- ✔ That the right payment allowances were applied

- ✔ That discounts were applied appropriately

- ✔ That no procedures were improperly denied

- ✔ If no payment was received, whether it was due to the entire amount being applied to the patient's deductible, the claim being denied, or some other reason

If anything is amiss — the payment allowances aren't correct, for example, or a procedure that should have approved was denied — then you need to appeal the claim and provide medical records and other necessary documentation to support your claim. Head to Chapter 14 for more on making an appeal.

## Meshing the COB with the EOB

Your EOB may address something known as *coordination of benefits* (COB), which has to do with benefits assigned to dependents or children who are covered under both their parents' insurance. If, for example, both parents are employed and have benefits, either one or both of the parents will have dependent coverage on the children. When both parents exercise this option, confusion often ensues. Here are some of the key issues that arrive with COB claims:

- ✔ When both parents exercise this option, whose plan is the *primary payer* (the first payer to be responsible for claim processing)? This is decided by *the birthday rule,* which states that the parent with the earlier birthday (by month and day, not year) is the primary payer. So if Mom's birthday is January 6 and Dad's birthday is May 31, Mom's insurance is the primary payer.

✔ If a claim is submitted to Dad's insurance when Mom's plan is the primary payer, what happens? Dad's insurance usually denies payment as the responsibility of another payer. If you submitted the claim to Dad's insurance after Mom's insurance paid, you also need to submit the EOB from Mom's insurance along with the claim to show that the claim was paid or priced by the correct payer.

Dealing with two-parent or dual coverage of an adolescent gets more complicated when a divorce is a factor in determining responsibility. Some divorce decrees assign responsibility for medical coverage to a certain parent, and this decree may conflict with the birthday rule. When this happens, getting the claim paid correctly takes tenacity, and you may need assistance from the parent(s). Similarly, when a responsible parent remarries and that spouse or step-parent becomes the primary carrier, getting claims paid correctly can take months.

✔ What happens if, for some reason, the primary payer's plan no longer insures the child? In this case, the parents need to contact the correct payer and update the records so that the claim will pay correctly. (**Note:** You can prevent this situation by verifying at check-in whether the insurance is the primary payer; refer to Chapter 11 for information on the kinds of things to check during check-in.)

## Dealing with subrogation

Insurance companies do not want to pay claims for which they are not responsible. There may be times that the patient's insurance pays the claim, then subrogates the claim with another company after determining that responsibility is that of another payer. *Subrogation* happens when a third party takes on the responsibility of another's legal right to collect the payment, which means that company A paid the original claim and then went to company B (maybe a homeowner's insurance) and asked to be reimbursed. When this happens, you may see an EOB come across your desk that shows the claim reversed but still paid.

Subrogation can be financially advantageous to a third-party payer who bears financial responsibility because it allows the non-contracted third party to benefit from the contracted pricing. After all, the third-party is simply reimbursing the amount the insurance company paid, which, because of contracted discounts and fee schedules, may be much less than a non-contracted payer would otherwise pay. The end result is usually a huge savings on claim settlement.

# Chapter 14

# Handling Disputes and Appeals

## In This Chapter

▶ Resolving disputes

▶ Knowing when an appeal is necessary

▶ Crafting an appeal that gets results

▶ Handling Medicare appeals

*F*iling that first claim is a great feeling. High fives all around. But just when you thought your job was done, you realize it's only just begun. After you master the front-of-house operations, you're ready to button things up on the back end, which, in the claim cycle, refers to following up outstanding claims and is just an insider's way of saying *collections*. At this point, you also may find yourself dealing with disputes with the payers. Maybe the payer didn't process the claim correctly. Maybe it denied payment entirely. In either case, your job is to figure out the cause of the dispute and work to resolve it. In this chapter, I tell you everything you need to know about the appeals process.

## Dealing with Disputes Involving Contract and Non-Contracted Payers

Most, if not all, disputes arise when the provider, your employer, is underpaid. Ideally, payer contracts clearly define a firm payment structure. Often, these contracts are based on Medicare fees, and as long as you're participating in the patient's plan, all is good. Sometimes a contracted payer processes a claim incorrectly, a kind of dispute that is easily remedied. Other types of disputes require more work. In the following sections, I explain what you can expect when handling disputes involving both contract and non-contracted payers.

 You can prevent many issues by verifying the patient's coverage prior to the encounter. Some plans require that certain procedures be authorized prior to being performed, for example; other plans (HMOs especially) may require a referral from the primary care physician before seeing a specialist. When you verify coverage, make sure you understand what, exactly, has been approved.

A referral may be just for a visit, for example, and if surgery or another procedure is deemed necessary, the patient may need another referral to be treated. So check because a little effort on the front end may save a lot of effort on the back end.

## Contract payers

Contract payers are those with whom your provider has a contract or who are part of a network with which the provider has a contract. The contract identifies the payment structure for each procedure and defines such issues as the following:

✔ The number of procedures that are to be paid per service date

✔ The reduction formula, often referred to as the multiple procedure reduction

With *multiple procedure reduction* (MPD), the first procedure is paid at 100 percent of contractual allowance; the second may be paid at a reduced rate, often 50 percent; and the third at whatever percentage is deemed appropriate per the contract. Medicare sets the standard by stating that the first procedure is paid at 100 percent and additional procedures are paid at 50 percent of the allowance. Some payers reduce subsequent procedures to 25 percent of the allowed amount, and others may limit the number of procedures that will be paid.

✔ Other payment guidelines, such as revenue code allowances, implant allowances (implants are plates, screws, anchors, and other hardware used to secure orthopedic repairs)

✔ The timely filing limit (Medicare is 180 days, but many commercial payers are less)

✔ The appeals process

If a payer fails to pay a claim as defined by contract, the appeals process is pretty simple: You simply write a letter that details the way the claim should have paid according to the contract. If the claim didn't pay as expected due to an ambiguity in the contract, you need to outline your expectations, refer to the contract, and stand firm. A well-structured contract averts any ambiguous processing.

## Non-contracted payers

Non-contracted payers are those with whom the provider does not have a contract. Payment for these claims is what is known as *out-of-network*, and you need to carefully investigate them prior to any patient encounter because some plans don't allow for out-of-network services.

Plans that don't allow payment for out-of-network providers may process the claim to make the entire billed amount the patient's responsibility, or they may pay the claim without applying a discount. Often, if a provider doesn't participate in a certain network, the payer negotiates through a third-party pricing agent and tries to obtain a discount from the provider. Other times, if a provider contacts an out-of-network payer prior to a patient encounter, the payer asks for a one-time agreement for payment.

In cases where the payer denies payment and the plan provisions stipulate that the patient is responsible for all charges, most providers try to work with the insurance company to get the claim paid. Therefore, before sending the patient a bill, try to talk to the patient's insurer to find out whether the issue can be resolved. You also want to let the patient know that her insurer has denied payment and see whether either she or her employer can assist in resolving the issue.

When you deal with non-contracted payers, you need to rely on correct claims processing guidelines (published by the Centers for Medicare & Medicaid Services [CMS]) and the pre-encounter verification. Commercial payers can always cry "NCCI edits" when processing an out-of-network claim. After that, they are bound by the provisions of the patient's coverage plan.

Patients are responsible for ensuring that any medical provider they seek treatment from accepts their insurance. However, the provider has a moral obligation, whenever possible, to verify patients' coverage prior to treating them.

# Knowing When to File an Appeal: General Guidelines

After you submit a claim to the payer, you can reasonably expect a response within 60 days. Often, larger payers respond within 15 days. If everything goes the way it should, the payer processes the claim as you anticipated, and the payment is correct. If either of these two things doesn't happen, you need to follow up.

## When general follow-up doesn't yield a timely payment

Following up may be as simple as calling the payer to see whether the claim has been received and where it stands in the adjudication process. (*Adjudication* refers to the payment obligation outlined in the patient's insurance benefits with regard to a claim.) Sometimes, the claim just isn't there, and you need to resubmit it and start the calendar again. Other times, the payer may need additional information from your office, another provider, or the patient.

If the payer needs information from your office, you can provide it simply enough. If he needs info from another provider, you may need to contact that other provider to see whether the payer's request has been received and whether the provider has responded. If information is needed from the patient, you probably need to contact the patient and ask her to contact her insurance company. If a claim does not pay as obligated by contract, you need to start the appeals process, explained in the section "Going through an Appeal, Step by Step."

## When mix-ups in accounts receivable result in a delay

Accounts receivable (AR) is the industry name for outstanding payments. All companies monitor how many days their numerous accounts have been in AR. For most companies, 90 days is tolerable, but going beyond that gets undesired attention from above. Outstanding AR can be a result of a slow payer, and most contracts contain language that obligates payment within a certain time. Many states have prompt pay statutes aimed at preventing claim stalling.

Often the cause of a high number of accounts receivable days is that the payer has not paid as expected. Claims processors use claim adjudication software to price claims. For payment to occur in a timely manner, the correct contract must be loaded for each claim. Sometimes, that doesn't happen, and the claim doesn't process according to contract. At that point, you must appeal the claim.

## The Art of the Appeal: What You Need to Know before You Begin

Preparing an appeal to correct an incorrectly processed claim is an art. You have to know enough about the details of the claim and the individual quirks of the payer to find a workable, timely solution. In the case of an appeal, the burden of proof is on the provider to show why the claim has not processed correctly.

How you approach an appeal has a big impact on how smoothly and quickly the process goes. In the following sections, I explain how to approach an appeal so that you maximize your chances of getting the reimbursement the provider is entitled to.

An appeal that is based on the contract and that clearly defines how the claim should have processed usually results in a reprocessed claim, especially if the contract has a prompt pay clause. If the payer failed to process the claim according to the contract and the error resulted in a delay of prompt payment, the payer may have to pay interest on the late dollars. Because this kind of error can cost payers a lot of money, they want the error fixed as much as you do.

## Knowing who you're dealing with

The primary contact between a provider and a payer is the provider representative. In most cases, however, your first point of contract is actually with the provider relations department, otherwise known as *provider services*. If you are responsible for claim follow-up, prepare to spend a lot of time on the phone with these individuals.

### Provider services

The people who work in provider services can check to see whether a claim was received, can usually provide a processing time, and can sometimes facilitate correcting an improperly processed claim. When a claim processing is not in compliance with the payer contract, often the remedy is a simple phone call. If the payer has loaded the contract correctly (refer to the earlier section "When mix-ups in accounts receivable result in a delay"), the provider services representative can identify the problem — usually with coaching from you — and send the claim back to processing with instructions regarding what needs to be done.

If your contract was not loaded correctly, then calls to provider services for resolution are useless because these representatives rely on the information loaded into their systems, and they have no way to verify contract specifics. In this case, you need to turn to your provider representative.

### Provider representative

If your contract wasn't loaded correctly, you address the problem through your provider representative, who is the individual responsible for making sure that the contract between the payer and the provider has been correctly loaded into the payer claims processing system(s).

In this situation, you need to contact the provider representative to let him know that the claims are not paying as agreed. Normally, you can get the name of the provider representative from the provider relations department or the payer website.

Your provider representative generally tries to assist with contract or claims issues, particularly issues that may cause several claims to pay incorrectly for the same reason — which is usually a contract problem. If you have a contract with the insurance company, disputes should be easily resolved. Without a contract, things can get difficult, so be sure to have all of your *i*'s dotted and *t*'s crossed.

## Knowing what to say and what not to say

During the appeal process, you want to keep to the facts. If a contract exists, refer to the language of the contract. If the problem is a bundling issue (one or more of the CPT codes on the claim are considered incidental or inclusive to another; refer to Chapter 4 or 12), then describe the extra work — be sure to include the extra time involved — and why this time investment was necessary. In addition, let the payer know what payment you are expecting or what payment agreement will be acceptable to close the claim.

Keep your emotions in check in these situations. The old saying that you can catch more flies with honey than vinegar totally applies here. Try to keep your comments positive and use appropriate, formal language on the phone and in written communications. Some effective phrases to use during appeals include:

- ✔ **"Our contract obligates CPT 5555 to allow $1,234."** Say this if you didn't receive the amount you should have or the payer disputes the amount owed.

- ✔ **"This service was authorized prior to the date of service by ABC, and this is the authorization number: 1234."** Say this when you want the claim to be reprocessed because it was denied for lack of precertification. (But make sure the correct procedural code was authorized! For more on prior authorizations, refer to Chapter 11.)

- ✔ **"We are aware of the edits; however, this procedure should not bundle because it required access through a separate incision."** This provides an explanation for your request for extra reimbursement.

- ✔ **"I can send a written appeal. Can you provide a fax number and address please?"** This information ensures that the claim gets to the right place.

- ✔ **"What do I need to do to facilitate this issue?"** or **"Who should I speak with about this problem?"** These questions alert the person on the other end that you plan to do what needs to be done to resolve the claim.

Avoid using phrases such as "It's not fair" or "We didn't know the surgery wasn't covered." Here's a newsflash: The payer doesn't care. Payers are running a business, and disputes regarding payment are just that — business — which is what they should be to you, too. So follow the payer's lead and keep things professional.

## Using the resources at your disposal

When you're appealing a claim, your primary resource is right in your filing cabinet or on your hard drive: It's your payer contracts. If, for example, a contract obligates claim payment of a certain amount, you would word you appeal to remind the payer of the contractual obligation: Basically, Payer XYZ agreed in the contract to pay $1,000 for procedure 23456 but paid only $700. Pretty straightforward stuff. A reminder of the contract should be all you need to have the situation corrected.

Other resources include the National Correct Coding Initiative (NCCI) edits, professional newsletters, and CPT assistant and numerous other coding guidelines. *Note:* Many specialties have published payment rules that may be different than the NCCI edits. Therefore, if your provider is a specialist, you can use this documentation to reference reasons for demanding that the claim be processed differently. Whatever specialty newsletters or coding guidelines you reference, if possible, send the written documentation with any appeals.

Although NCCI edits are the most widely recognized, other editing systems exist. Look in the contracts to see which edits a payer follows, and verify which edits were followed when processing the claim[s].

# Going through an Appeal, Step by Step

When a claim does not pay as accepted, the first course of action is normally a phone call. Ask the representative whether the issue can be resolved; if not, seek direction to initiate the appeal or reconsideration process. If you're dealing with a commercial payer, the payer may have a reconsideration form on its website that providers can use to challenge a payment decision. If not, then the formal written appeals process begins. The next sections take you through these steps.

## Making the initial call

In most cases, the most efficient first step in the appeals process is to make a phone call to the payer. Writing letters takes time, and then it takes even more time for the recipient to read the letter, verify the argument, and then forward the claim to be corrected. If the problem is simple, you may be able to have the claim sent back simply by calling the payer. (For more complicated issues, you may need to begin with a letter; head to the next section for details about these situations.)

Before discussing the claim with you, the provider representative — the person employed by the payer to work with you regarding disputes —verifies your need to know. Expect the representative to ask for the following information:

- ✔ Your name.
- ✔ The name of your company and tax ID number or the NPI (National Provider Identifier) number.

   The NPI is the ten digit number required by HIPAA (Health Insurance Portability and Accountability Act) to identify providers in electronic transactions.
- ✔ The patient's ID (the identification number assigned by the payer), name, and date of birth.
- ✔ The date of service in question.
- ✔ The billed amount of the claim. (This is the dollar total of the claim, not what you are expecting to be paid.)

After you verify your need to know, you have the opportunity to tell the provider representative why the claim has not processed correctly. Often the representative can look at the claim, look at your contract, and verify what needs to be done. If that happens, the representative can usually send the claim back to the processor with instructions to reprocess. Sometimes, the phone call alone may be enough to resolve the issue. If it's not, you need to follow up with a letter, as the next section explains.

Make sure you document all phone conversations in the patient system or billing software. Note who you spoke with, what the agreement was, and the reference number (get this number from the provider representative; it documents the conversation on the payer's end). This kind of documentation is essential when a potential filing issue arises.

## *It's in the mail: Composing an appeal letter*

Sometimes, a phone call just isn't enough. The issue may be complicated and easier to document in writing. For example:

✔ If the problem is a bundling issue, a written appeal is always necessary. You can't argue unbundling without supplying the documentation that supports the request for additional payment.

✔ If you are dealing with a third-party pricing issue, you may need to send a letter to the payer and the third-party pricing agent.

✔ If taking legal action becomes necessary, you need the written proof of your attempt to secure correct payment.

### What to include in your letter

In your appeal letter, be sure to include the claim number, patient name and ID number, the date of service, and the amount billed.

Begin the body of the letter by outlining your expectations for claim settlement. Then explain why the claim should pay per the expectations you describe. After that, reiterate your expectations, including the time frame that payment is expected and the follow-up action you'll take if the claim doesn't reprocess as you've outlined. Figures 14-1 and 14-2 show requests for reconsideration, one for a contracted payer, the other for a non-contracted payer.

Be prepared to follow through on any implied actions. If you say that the matter will be referred to your attorney in 30 days, then send it as promised. Similarly, if you say that the issue will be sent to the insurance commission in 30 days, do it.

### Using reconsideration request forms

Some commercial payers or insurance companies have something called *reconsideration request forms* available on their websites. That's just a fancy way of saying "claims form," but you get the picture. Depending upon the company's preferences, you can submit some forms online; others must be mailed or faxed.

These standard forms are for simple appeals — called *first-level appeals* — that are contractually based and need very little argument. If this initial appeal is denied, you need to file a formal second-level appeal, which is a letter that outlines your request and the reason for your position along with the supporting documentation. (You can read more about the different levels of appeals in the section "Maxing out your appeals.")

April 10, 2012

Global Health United
12345 Business Parkway
Bigtown, TX 54321

Claim appeal – Or Request for reconsideration

RE:   Patient Name: John Q. Public
      ID (or Claim) #: 55555
      Service Date: 2-1-2012
      Billed Charges: $1,200.00

To Whom It May Concern:

The above claim was not processed correctly. Our contract obligates this
claim to be paid as follows:

CPT 12345 is obligated to pay $1,000 per contract. This amount is due at
100% of obligation. CPT 78901 is obligated at 50% of the $400 contractual
obligation, or $200.

Please verify the above in our contract and reprocess correctly. If I can be of
further assistance, please do not hesitate to contact me between the hours of
8AM and 5PM CST at (555) 555- 5555.

Respectfully,

Mary Smith, CPC

**Figure 14-1:**
A request
for recon-
sideration
for a
contracted
payer.

### Other stuff to know about sending an appeal letter

When you send an appeal, keep the following points in mind:

✔ Notify the intermediary, if one was involved, that the payer has refused
to honor the negotiated settlement.

March 13, 2012

Global Health United
12345 Business Parkway
Bigtown, TX 54321

RE:  Claim number: 123456789
     Patient Name: Jane Doe
     ID Number: 55555
     Service Date: 2-1-2012
     Billed Charges: $1,234.00

To Whom It May Concern:

The above referenced claim was not paid correctly. We do not have a contract that obligates us to accept this discount. Please identify the contract accessed when pricing this claim, along with documentation that supports any association with that contract to this provider. If no contract was utilized, then please identify the methodology used to price this claim.

Stall tactics such as this that delay correct claims processing is a violation of Indiana Statute 987 and as such will be reported to the State Insurance Commissioner thirty days from the date of this notice if the issue is not promptly resolved to our satisfaction.

We will settle this claim upon receipt of $1,110.06, which represents 90% of billed charges.

Sincerely,


XYZ Billing and Coding

On behalf of Dr. Jones

**Figure 14-2:**
A request
for recon-
sideration
for a non-
contracted
payer.

✔ Prior to sending the appeal, call the payer to verify where the appeal should be sent. If the claim was priced by a network and paid by a commercial payer, send the appeal to both and let them know that each has been notified of the payment deficiency.

✔ Check to see whether the network priced the claim or whether the payer simply accessed the network itself.

# Back on the phone again: Following up when the check doesn't arrive

If the appealed claim does not bear fruit in the form of a check, you may start to get a little nervous. At this point, put on your happy voice and call for a follow-up to check on the status of the check. When you do speak with a payer, just as when you compose the appeal letter, always base your argument or appeal on facts found in contracts, agreements, professional publications, and your resources about medical necessity.

Always be clear with regard to the reason for your call and have all of the necessary information at hand. You need the provider's NPI number and/or tax ID number. The payer uses these numbers to verify your identity and that you have a right to make the inquiry. You also need the patient's ID number, his or her date of birth, the date of service, and the billed amount of the claim (the total dollar amount).

Fully document all conversations with payers or patients in the patient record, which is usually part of the billing software. Clearly state what was said and by whom, and get the name of the person with whom you are speaking.

In the following sections, I list the kinds of questions and information you should gather. In all these cases, verify how long resolving the issue will take and set up a tickler system to remind yourself, or your staff, to follow up if that date passes and the issue hasn't been resolved as promised. Base your timing for the next follow-up call on the feedback from the representative. But always check at least every 30 days on all outstanding claims.

A *tickler system* gives unprompted reminders. You can use a calendar, as long as you can remember to look at it. Even better, if your office uses a program like Microsoft Outlook or Gmail, you can set up these automatic reminders in the system's calendar, and they'll pop up on the appointed date and time.

### Asking general follow-up questions

When following up with payers, ask the following questions and document the answers in the file:

✔ **When was the claim received?** Don't assume the claim reached its destination. Each lost claim is lost revenue. Therefore, within 30 days of initial claims submission, make sure you follow up with the insurance companies to verify that the claim was received and is in process. After the 30-day deadline, the next deadline is 90 days. Any claim that is 90 days old needs to be investigated.

✔ **Has the claim been assigned a claim number? If so, what is it?** Make a note of this number.

✔ **Is any additional documentation needed to complete the claim processing?** If additional information is requested, make arrangements to submit that information. After you send it, follow up in a week or 10 days to make sure that the claim is again in process.

✔ **What is the anticipated completion date for the processing?** Make a note of this date; payment should follow.

✔ **What is the reference number for this call and the name of the person with whom you're speaking?** This information lets you document all calls going forward.

### Questions to ask if the rep tells you that the claim has been paid

If the representative tells you that the claim has been paid, ask these questions:

✔ What is the check number?

✔ What is the allowed amount of the claim? If the allowed amount is not correct, ask the representative whether the claim can be sent back for correct processing. Repeat the obligation as defined in the contract and restate why the allowance is incorrect.

✔ What is the amount of the check?

✔ Does the patient have any responsibility for claim payment, such as copay, co-insurance, or unmet deductible?

✔ When was the check sent?

✔ Where was the check sent?

✔ What is the reference number for the call? Document this in the billing software.

### Questions to ask when the claim hasn't been paid as expected

If you are calling because a claim has not paid as expected, note the following:

✔ Why the claim processed the way it did.

If a contract was utilized and pricing was incorrect, notify the representative of the correct obligation according to your records.

✔ The claim editing software that was utilized to process the claim.

✔ The correct address to send a written appeal. (Also, note the account and keep a copy.)

✔ The representative you're speaking to.

## Maxing out your appeals

In a perfect world, claims always get paid on the first go-round. And if a claim does not pay correctly at first, you can either call or send a written appeal, and the payer will recognize his error and process the claim correctly. Alas, we don't live in a perfect world. Sometimes, even after the phone call and letter, the claim still isn't processed. In that case, you need to follow the appeals process as outlined in your contract.

Some payer contracts outline their appeals process. Several define the process in steps such as first-level appeal, second-level appeal, and request for outside review as the final level. I explain these levels in the next sections.

When sending a written appeal, whether it's a first- or second-level appeal, send medical records and a copy of the claim along with a copy of the explanation of benefits (EOB) that was included with the payment. The EOB shows how the claim payment was calculated. Including the EOB helps the payer identify the claim, including the individual processor. If you don't include a copy, make sure that the claim number is on the appeal so that the payer can identify the correct claim.

### First-level appeals

A first-level appeal may just be a reminder that, according to your records, the claim should have processed a certain way. It's basically a friendly reminder that the contract wasn't followed or a discount was applied without a contract. If the problem is purely a pricing issue, this reminder may be all you need, and the payer will correct the error without further delay.

If the problem is that the claim was denied for medical necessity or anything of that nature, include all documentation with your first-level appeal. When you do so, the payer (hopefully) will reverse its decision and reprocess the claim correctly. If your first-level appeal defines the reason for the request along with any supporting documentation, it may be the only appeal you need.

The response time to appeals is often included in your contract and varies among payers. In cases where the payer has implemented new processing software and has multiple claims paying incorrectly (or not at all), the backlog can quickly become months. If you have not had a reply within 30 days, follow up to make sure that the appeal has been received. Each state has its own prompt payment statute, so your timing also depends on the statutes for your individual state.

### Second-level appeals

Sometimes, the payer denies your request. In this case, you need to send another request. The second request is called a *second-level appeal.* You may need to send this appeal to a different address, or you may be able to simply mark it "second level" in order to identify that you have asked for resolution once already.

A second-level appeal is more formal. In it, make sure you do the following:

- ✔ **Clearly define the problem and note that you have asked once already without success.** You may even include a copy of your original appeal.

   In a second-level appeal, if you can state your case in a different way, try to do so. Sometimes simply rephrasing your words makes a huge difference in the success of a second-level appeal.

- ✔ **Include all documentation.** This documentation would include things like the EOB, medical records, applicable invoices, and a copy of the contract (or the applicable section of the contract). (**Note:** If you send a copy of the claim, make sure to mark it "COPY.")

Check your contract before sending a second-level appeal. Some payer contracts specify that the second-level appeal is the final level, and if it is denied, no further appeal options are possible. In this case, check your contract for options. The contract may identify a third-party mediation process for disputes if the dollar value is high enough. If you're dealing with a non-contracted payer, you can involve an attorney. Most offices have an attorney who specializes in healthcare and can handle the matter for you.

# Appealing Medicare Processing

The Centers for Medicare & Medicaid Services (CMS) has a defined process for appealing. This process is easy to follow and quite efficient. You can find all the necessary forms on the Medicare website (www.medicare.gov) and individual contracted Medicare carrier websites.

The preferred method for submission is online. You can also submit additional documentation as well. The Medicare online appeal site provides a cover sheet that you can use to mail or fax the documentation to the appropriate address for consideration.

Medicare tends to see everything as black and white and makes all decisions based on the policies that were in effect on the service date. So as long as you or your software stays current with regard to Medicare policy, then appealing to this payer is quite painless.

In the following sections, I take you through the Medicare appeals process.

## Request for redetermination

The request for redetermination is a friendly reminder that the Medicare processing does not reflect the local fee schedule. You can find the initial request form at www.medicare.gov. Most Local Coverage Carriers or Medicare contractors have links to this form on their individual websites, and many allow the appeal to be submitted online with supporting documents faxed, using the assigned cover sheet.

My advice is to submit online if possible to avoid any potential timely appeal issues. According to Medicare rules, an appeal must be submitted within 90 days of the initial determination. If you submit online, you have proof of timely submission.

If the contractor doesn't grant your request or provide solid evidence that the claim has already processed correctly, the next level of appeal is to a Qualified Independent Contractor.

## Qualified Independent Contractor (QIC) reconsideration

If your request for redetermination doesn't resolve the problem, next up is the Qualified Independent Contractor (QIC) reconsideration. You must submit this request within 180 days of the receipt of your redetermination reply. The instructions for submitting this appeal are on the redetermination notice. With this form, you can also submit additional evidence.

The QIC is the last level of appeal that allows you to submit additional evidence, but the best approach is to submit *all* evidence with the initial request for redetermination. When you submit evidence later, you have to include with the evidence an explanation as to why you didn't submit it with the original request and why it's now relevant.

To file a QIC, you must use the reconsideration request form (CMS-20033) which you can find on the CMS website (www.cms.gov/Medicare/CMS-Forms/CMS-Forms). If you choose not to use this form, be sure to include the following information on your request:

- ✔ Beneficiary (patient) name and Medicare number.
- ✔ The specific service(s) or item(s) for which the reconsideration is being requested, along with the date of service.

✔ The name and signature of the provider. As the representative of the provider, you use your name and sign the form.

✔ The name of the Medicare contractor who made the redetermination. To save time, you also want to include a copy of the redetermination.

✔ An explanation why you still disagree with the processing.

✔ Any additional evidence, along with explanations for why you didn't submit this information earlier and why it's relevant now. (Medicare may exclude evidence that has been submitted late unless you can show good cause for submitting it late.)

The QIC written decision is normally received within 60 days and contains an explanation of the ruling and information regarding whether an additional level of appeal is available. The next level is to take your appeal to an Administrative Law Judge. Additional evidence is not allowed at the upper level of appeal unless you have a documented reason why the evidence was not previously submitted.

## Administrative Law Judge Hearing (ALJ)

If you are not satisfied by the two previous levels of appeal, then you may request an Administrative Law Judge hearing. You can find the necessary form (everything requires a form!) at www.medicare.gov. But you can also present your case in writing. In this request, outline the area in dispute, along with the case number assigned by the QIC, the Medicare number of the patient, the original claim number assigned by the Medicare contract, and all evidence previously submitted. You must also identify the claims processing rules that support your request and the reason you feel the process has not been followed.

Currently the amount in dispute must be a minimum of $130 before an ALJ hearing can be requested. This amount may increase annually based on the consumer price index.

When conducting a claims review, the judge conducts a hearing, reviews all the evidence, and makes a decision based upon Medicare rules and the law. Most hearings are held via videoconference or telephone, although you may request a hearing in person. The judge decides whether a hearing of this type is warranted. You may also request that the judge make a decision without a hearing, based solely upon the written evidence submitted. Medicare and its contractors are also notified of the hearing and are allowed to participate.

Hearings are conducted in person and over the phone. You may also request that the ALJ review the evidence and make a ruling. In a hearing, both parties are entitled to attend, although Medicare usually declines and leaves the decision in the hands of the ALJ. The burden of proof is on the provider. For this reason, some providers rely on legal representation if the amount in question is large. The ALJ level of appeal is not for the novice.

The ALJ normally makes a decision within 90 days, although this time frame is often extended for several reasons, including a heavier than normal caseload and evidence being submitted late.

If your claim is denied by the ALJ and you still feel that your claim has been processed incorrectly, the next level of appeal is the Medicare Appeals Council.

The Office of Medicare Hearings and Appeals (OMHA) was created by the Medicare Modernization Act of 2003. The purpose of this office is to streamline the appeals process and make it more efficient. The people in this office include a Chief Administrative Law Judge and the regional or Associate Chief Administrative Law Judges, each of whom has an assistant known as the Hearing Office Director. OMHA is responsible for the level-three Medicare appeals process.

## *Medicare Appeals Council (MAC) and Judicial Review*

The Medicare Appeals Council (MAC) is part of the Departmental Appeals Board of the Department of Health & Human Services (HHS). It is independent of the other appeal boards.

To submit a request, you use form DAB-101, which you can download from the Health & Human Services website (www.hhs.gov). You can either submit the appeal online (doing so requires that you register with the Departmental Appeals Board electronic filing system on the HHS website), or you can submit a request in writing.

Make sure the written request includes the following:

- ✔ Beneficiary (patient) name and Medicare number.
- ✔ The specific service(s) or item(s) for which the reconsideration is being requested, along with the date of service.

✔ The date of the ALJ decision and a copy of the decision.

✔ The name and signature of the provider. As the representative of the provider, you use your name and sign the form.

After you complete the form, you can fax it to (202) 565-0227 or mail it to the following address:

Department of Health & Human Services
Departmental Appeals Board
Medicare Appeals Council, MS 6127
Cohen Building Room G-644
330 Independence Ave., S.W.
Washington, D.C. 20201

You must file the appeal within 60 days after receiving the ALJ's decision. The MAC assumes that you received the decision five days after the date on decision itself. Therefore, timeliness is a huge factor, and if your appeal is late, you need good cause.

The MAC may dismiss, deny, or grant your request. It also has the option of returning the issue back to the ALJ for reconsideration. Most providers opt not to pursue the Medicare Appeals Council level.

If the reimbursement amount in question is above the current minimum requirement (it changes annually), then the next level of appeal is by Judicial Review in a Federal District Court. The notice received from the MAC provides information needed to file a civil action, which represents the final level of appeal. At this level, the provider will benefit by using an attorney, and the legal costs will likely outweigh any perceived wrongs.

# Appealing a Workers' Comp Claim

Often an out-of-network payer is responsible for paying a Workers' Compensation claim. Many states have legislation in place or fee schedules that outline how Workers' Compensation claims will be paid. Other carriers participate in networks that offer pricing for these claims. Some organizations, referred to as *silent PPOs,* price claims for carriers who don't have a contract with the service provider as though the provider participates in the network. The provider has the right to fight these discounts.

Workers' Compensation claims demand up-front work. Someone in the provider's office should be responsible for verifying benefits, and this person should also verify the Workers' Compensation eligibility of the patient prior to any procedure being performed. (Coders are very good at verifying benefits because they have a thorough understanding of planned procedures and supporting diagnosis codes.)

Each Workers' Compensation patient has a caseworker, who is usually the coordinator for medical care, and this caseworker's name appears on any paperwork you receive. When dealing with Workers' Comp, you also work with an adjuster, who is responsible for coordinating the provider claims. Most Workers' Compensation claims have a set amount that has been approved to pay for medical expenses related to the worker's injury. The adjuster keeps track of these funds as they are paid out and may need to go back to the carrier or employer and ask for additional funds (if any are available). Get the adjuster's name up front and give him a call to make sure that you know where to send the claim and what additional documentation you must submit.

In addition to communicating with the caseworker and adjuster, you also want to verify the claim number, date of injury, and the body part that relates to the claim. Many carriers also require that all claims be submitted with the approved diagnosis code, so make sure that you and your employer know what diagnosis is covered.

When the claim is paid other than expected, referencing a network with which the provider is not familiar and taking a discount that the provider has not agreed to, then the appeals process begins. Often these underpriced claims are sent to the provider's attorney for a fair settlement. Depending on the office structure, the office manager or administrator is usually the one who sends the claim to the company attorney for action.

# Chapter 15

# Keeping Up with the Rest of the World

*M*any parts of your job, particularly those that involve codes, coding software, and procedures, are established and maintained by large organizations. One of the biggest of these is the World Health Organization (WHO), an organization that evaluates and responds to world health trends. The coding standards you must adhere to play a large role in how WHO accomplishes its mission, because it uses these codes to amass data on what's going on in the world. And where do these all-important codes come from? The international classifications of disease (ICD), the common system of codes that, up until this point, you may have thought had no other purpose than to overwhelm you with a zillion technical-sounding acronyms.

As a biller/coder, you play a key role in helping these professional governing bodies keep everything on the up-and-up and collect data that impacts just about every decision made in the healthcare field, from how to improve coding functions to what to spend research dollars on.

In this chapter, I explain how the healthcare industry is moving toward being more specific when reporting diagnosis codes that support medical necessity, the players involved with that big change, and how it will affect you.

# Who's WHO and Why You Should Care

You already know that your job as a biller/coder is to capture all billable procedures from the medical record and to make sure that each procedure you bill has a diagnosis code that documents medical necessity and justifies the procedure being billed. (If you don't know this already, read all about it in Part II.) But what you may not know yet is that the information you communicate from the provider to the payer is also submitted to the information gathering organization known as the World Health Organization (WHO).

WHO is the United Nations organization that views disease and injury from a world perspective and uses the data it gathers on world health trends to recommend the direction of (or need for) research based on its findings. WHO is responsible for coordinating leadership and providing direction on global public health issues by setting standards for healthcare documentation and monitoring health trends.

WHO makes identifying, monitoring, and containing infectious disease outbreaks (like the HIV/AIDS outbreak) possible at the international level, which has resulted in millions of saved lives. WHO has also been instrumental in the development and distribution of drugs, vaccines, and other disease-fighting efforts. The United States is one of almost 200 countries that is member to this organization.

When it was founded in 1948, the original purpose of WHO was to identify methods that would provide better health to people worldwide. This goal has led to standards for safe drinking water, better sanitation methods, access to vaccinations, free birth control, and programs to combat hunger. Following are some of WHO's primary goals today:

✔ Facilitating health development in impoverished areas, focusing specifically on chronic and tropical diseases

✔ Fostering health security, including preventing disease outbreaks and addressing epidemic threats

✔ Improving logistics, such as access to medicine, training medical staff, and helping more people access care

✔ Interpreting research for new policy ideas and organizing resources into collaborative efforts

Although WHO does not conduct research itself, it does support and coordinate research efforts throughout the world by arranging conferences that encourage collaboration among researchers worldwide.

## Helping the world's neediest cases

Monitoring the health of the entire globe is a big job, and WHO doesn't want to leave any country behind when it comes to disease management. That's why WHO works hard to provide healthcare access to underdeveloped countries. To address this need, WHO announced an agenda that challenged member countries to implement a system for a universal healthcare plan and to identify methods, such as increasing taxes and implementing improved budget guidelines, for raising funds to finance these healthcare plans.

WHO also encourages the improvement of healthcare in the most impoverished countries via providing access to primary care providers (preventative care reduces incidents of disease and allows for the treatment of minor illness before they can progress) and to prenatal care (to promote healthier pregnancies and

healthier babies and to reduce maternal mortality). Perhaps one of WHO's biggest challenges has been the fight against HIV/AIDS.

WHO has made Africa the focus of efforts to address current health issues like these. Why? Because Africa remains the continent with the highest incidence of diseases in the world. Despite awareness of the spread of HIV and AIDS, it is still the leading cause of death among the citizens of this continent. The statistics are staggering: As of 2009, the Joint United Nations Program on HIV/AIDS (UNAIDS) organization estimated that 22.5 million people in sub-Saharan Africa were afflicted with HIV. So, it's no wonder that WHO has made this disease, as well as the general health of developing countries, a very high priority.

WHO works very hard to keep the world population healthy. To do that, WHO needs the data you supply to be as specific as possible. As a coder, you are the individual responsible for abstracting the data that will eventually find its way into the WHO database.

# Charting Your Course with ICD

The international classification of diseases (most commonly known as ICD) classifies any disease or health problem you code. Basically, ICD is the common system of codes that you use everyday in your billing and coding work. Each diagnosis code provides a general description of the disease or injury that led to the patient/physician encounter.

ICD codes are divided into two categories:

- ✔ **ICD-CM (clinical modification):** Clinical modifications are diagnosis codes that all healthcare providers use.
- ✔ **ICD-PCS (procedure coding system):** The procedure codes are used only for inpatient reporting (hospital billing and coding).

These codes are not only used by billers and coders when they fill out claim forms, but they're used by others to classify diseases and other health problems on many types of health records, including death certificates, to help provide national mortality and morbidity rates.

WHO (which I discuss in the preceding section) uses the data gleaned from the codes you submit to analyze the health of large population groups and monitor diseases and other health problems for all members of our global community. For your purposes, you can think of the ICD codes as the language you speak to communicate with organizations like WHO so that they can keep the world healthy.

## Looking at the differences between ICD-9 to ICD-10

Repeat after me: ICD-9 is to ICD-10 as VCR is to DVR. In other words, ICD-9 is the old school coding classification system, while ICD-10 is the new kid in town.

The differences between the two are fairly significant. Here are a couple of areas where they differ:

- **Number of codes:** ICD-9 has just over 14,000 diagnosis codes and almost 4,000 procedural codes. In contrast, ICD-10 contains over 68,000 diagnosis codes (clinical modification codes) and over 72,000 procedural codes.

- **The info conveyed by the code:** ICD-9 codes contain three to five digits beginning with either a number or a letter, with a decimal point placed after the third digit, and the ICD-9 book indicates the level of specificity for each code. ICD-10 codes, on the other hand, are seven digits in length. The first three digits are similar to the corresponding ICD-9 code, with a decimal point after the third digit. But the digits that follow the decimal point have specific meaning. For medical and surgical procedures, for example, the digits that follow are specific to body part, surgical approach, and other qualifiers needed for billing. Similarly, the ICD-10 CM (clinical modification) codes that represent diagnosis codes also have seven digits (each digit is replaced by a place holder if it is not needed). The first three are similar to the ICD-9 code, but the additional codes add specificity to the code such as laterality, chronic versus acute, and so on.

The latest revision of ICD, ICD-10, has been in effect since 1998, but you wouldn't know that here in the U.S., which is the last industrialized nation to implement ICD-10 and has managed to stage a 10-year delay as it continues to use the 30-plus-year-old ICD-9 system. Opposition to ICD-10 is primarily based on the timing of initial costs (for things like reprogramming software and IT platforms and training all the personnel involved in medical billing or coding), particularly at a time when the U.S. is trying to control the rising cost of healthcare. Today, despite pushback from medical organizations like the American Medical Association (AMA), the United States is planning to go forward with ICD-10 implementation.

The move to ICD-10 involves more training for you because ICD-10 codes are all seven-character long alphanumeric codes. If a specific "place" in the code isn't to be used, a placeholder character (x) replaces it. This represents an entirely different way of coding and will challenge even the most seasoned professionals in the early stages.

## *Moving from ICD-9 to ICD-10*

The ninth edition of the ICD classification is ICD-9, which the U.S. has used since 1979. But ICD-10 is coming, ready or not. All healthcare providers are obligated to be ICD-10 ready by October 1, 2014. (This date may be delayed by the U.S. Department of Health & Human Services [HHS], but providers are advised to continue preparation.)

The ICD-10 codes will result in more specific data, which in turn will assist WHO in its effort to identify viral mutations and other health threats that may affect people all over the world.

Because getting everyone the world over ready for the change is such a gargantuan task, ICD-10 is being implemented in phases:

- ✓ **Phase 1:** Develop an implementation plan and identify the potential impact on various office operations

- ✓ **Phase 2:** Implement preparation, working with software vendors and clearinghouses to ensure compatibility

- ✓ **Phase 3:** Go live with 5010 platform (discussed in the next section) in preparation for ICD-10 file transfer

- ✓ **Phase 4:** Address and correct deficiencies identified in Phase 3

Educators and companies that publish coding materials have been working for several years to prepare coders like you for the transition. The AAPC (formerly the American Academy of Professional Coders) and the American Health Information Management Association (AHIMA) have sponsored and will continue to sponsor workshops to assist coders in this process. Be sure to check out these workshops. Both organizations will also implement an ICD-10 certification testing process.

## Working on the 5010 platform

Some of the transition stuff for ICD-10 happens on the tech end of things, particularly with the transmission platforms your coding software uses to push claims through to the clearinghouse. In preparation for ICD-10, providers, clearinghouses, and payers have transitioned to 5010 transmission platforms, the method of transmitting the claim files for payment to the insurance companies.

### Piece of (layer) cake? Not quite

Using the 5010 platform, claims are transmitted electronically, and information that is entered into the billing software is then sent to the clearinghouse. In this system, each part of the claim can be pictured as a layer (or level), like this:

- ✔ The first layer (or level) contains information about the patient.

- ✔ The second layer contains information about the procedures and diagnosis codes.

- ✔ The third layer contains payer-specific information: the payer name, payer ID number, patient ID number, group number, and so on.

- ✔ The fourth layer contains the provider information, including name, address, and National Provider Identification (NPI) number.

- ✔ The final layer is a view of the entire claim.

When a problem exists with the claim due to any of these transmission levels, the IT people fix it. All you can usually do as a coder is identify where in the claims process the problem may be. In other words, you'll need to have your IT person on speed dial!

Even though this all sounds a little complicated (and it is), jumping on the ICD-10 bandwagon is good for several reasons. Proponents of ICD-10 argue that the improved data you get from using the new 5010 platform and subsequent coding changes will ultimately reduce healthcare costs such that the ICD transition will pay for itself. ICD-10 documentation will result in greater specificity in patient medical records, which will assist in assessment of treatment risk and frequency of procedural complications. It may also make documenting medical necessity for certain treatments easier.

### Troubleshooting the 5010

Experts have already identified problems associated with the 5010 transition, the primary one being that providers aren't getting paid, or payments are vastly delayed. The transition has resulted in delayed claims processing and is causing the days in accounts receivable (AR) to grow.

The problem is that 5010 transmissions require electronic fields to populate differently than they did with the old platform, and some billing software systems aren't uploading as expected. The result? Claims are stalling at the clearinghouse. When a claim is delayed at the clearinghouse, you usually have to manually fix the error until the correct software patch has been identified.

Here are some signs you can look for that indicate your provider's 5010 claims have a problem:

- ✔ **You see an increase in rejections or claim denials.** The problem may be that the billing software the provider uses isn't sending the required information to the clearinghouse. Or it may be that the clearinghouse is not formatting the claim correctly before sending it on to the payer or intermediary. To get to the bottom of the problem as quickly as possible, give every rejection or denial top priority.

- ✔ **You're no longer getting payments or explanation of benefits (EOBs) from payers who make payments via electronic fund transfers.** The problem may be that the pay-to information isn't transmitting correctly. Find out where the payment is and why; then find out how to fix it. Perhaps during 5010 transition, the payer incorrectly loaded the provider information, or maybe the information isn't populating correctly on the outgoing claim.

- ✔ **Claims that used to automatically cross over (Medicare to secondary payers, for example) no longer cross.** Check to make sure that payers such as Medicare who cross claims automatically to a secondary payer are receiving the secondary information on the claim. Some payers also cross over when the patient has a primary and secondary plan with the same payer. If the automatic crossovers stop, call the primary payer and ask why the claim wasn't sent. If they sent it, call the secondary payer and see whether the claim was received. If not, investigate and find out why. The likely culprit is a missing field on the claim, or the intermediary may have left it out during primary submission.

- ✔ **Primary claims show that they were sent by the billing software, but the clearinghouse doesn't acknowledge receipt.** Check and compare batch reports daily to make sure each claim sent is acknowledged. If the claims go missing at the clearinghouse, check with the software vendor to make sure that the file is being created and that you are sending the right file. Some of the 5010 software systems create more than one batch, so you have to know which one to upload. The clearinghouse or software vendor should be able to help you identify which batch is the correctly formatted one.

The clearinghouse can fix some errors; for those the clearinghouse can't fix, you must identify errors and then implement the fix on your end. Either way, the claim is delayed.

Other delays can occur at the payer, whose software must be 5010 ready as well. Most payers conduct 5010 readiness drills in preparation for these submissions, but depending upon provider and clearinghouse software, the claims are still not loading correctly and require manual intervention, which again causes delay.

### Looking at possible reasons for claim denial under 5010

Every step that delays the claim also delays the payment. Possible causes of rejections or denials under 5010 include the following:

- **Failure to bill under the NPI number:** The old platform, 4010, allowed claims to be billed under the Tax ID number.

- **Using a P.O. box or an abbreviated zip code for the provider's address.** The 5010 platform requires a physical address to be provided as a place of service; a P.O. box is not acceptable. In addition, the zip code must be the full nine digits.

- **Exceeding the number of diagnosis codes a procedure can be linked to:** Each procedure can be linked to a maximum of four diagnosis codes if you submit it on an HCFA.

- **Not using verbal code descriptions when needed:** Unlisted or unspecified procedural codes must have a verbal code description.

- **Not including a secondary payer indicator when needed:** If Medicare is the primary payer and a secondary payer or supplement plan exists, the secondary payer indicator must be on the claim.

# Facilitating the Transition to ICD-10 in Your Own Office

The compliance deadline for 5010 was delayed, and the AMA is working hard to extend the deadline. The AMA is also working to delay the ICD-10 transition as well, but a practice with an eye on the future will continue to prepare for the transition to 5010 and, subsequently, ICD-10.

As you move toward ICD-10 (and you will!), remember that claim transactions are the foundation of the financial stability of every healthcare provider's practice, be it a physician or non-physician provider. You should still be ready for the transition and not risk the chance of being unable to file claims.

ICD-10 demands a transition plan both for the physician and his or her staff. To put it bluntly: Get ready! Discuss with your employer the training needed for each member of the staff and stress the need for further education, without which you (and the other office staff members) will struggle with choosing the correct codes and helping the physician and clinical staff improve the documentation techniques necessary for correct coding.

## *Laying the ICD-10 groundwork*

To make all of this ICD magic happen, your provider is going to have to update the office billing software (as will the clearinghouse and every payer). Providers should prepare for ICD-10 well before the implementation deadline, which means that you have some prep work to do as well. Here are some steps that can help you and your provider prepare for the big switch:

1. **Prepare a report that lists currently used ICD-9 codes in order of frequency.**

   Online tools or cross coding translators that map ICD-9 codes to ICD-10 codes can help with this task. (The AAPC has an ICD-10 code translator, and so does Medicare.) These can assist in identifying the ICD-10 codes that the provider will likely use the most.

2. **After you identify the most frequently used codes, check current documentation and see whether it supports the mapped codes.**

   If your office uses a super-bill, you can start with the ICD-9 codes that are listed on the form to identify the matching ICD-10 codes and make sure that current documentation supports the replacement codes. (***Note:*** Everyone on the coding and billing staff should also be prepared to learn these codes and the specific anatomical relationship each represents.)

3. **After you complete this exercise for the most frequently used codes, expand to the other specialized codes that pertain to the office clientele.**

   By completing Steps 1–3, you have identified the ICD-10 codes that will soon be part of the daily routine.

4. **Alert the practitioner to the specific documentation that is missing from current patient records.**

If the office will continue to use super-bills, this process can help identify which codes should be listed on the form. You can also work with the billing software vendor to make sure that the ICD-10 codes that are likely to be used immediately upon transition are programmed into the software. If not, you can make them aware of your expectations.

Getting your software vendor involved with the switch is just as important as doing the necessary work on your end, so make sure that your software vendor is able to meet the new office needs and is willing to give you all planned updates along with transition dates and deadlines in writing.

## Prepping the office staff

After the back end is ready to roll for ICD-10 (things like software), then you can begin to prepare yourself and your colleagues for the daily details of how the new coding platform will change the way you all work. Consider the following examples of changes you'll see:

- **ICD-10 certification will require a more thorough understanding of human anatomy and physiology.** If you already struggle with assignment of ICD-9 codes, you'll want to brush up on what you know about the body.

- **With regard to coding and documentation purposes, prepare to be more specific in your coding.** This increased specificity means that you'll have to gather more information when you're conducting a physician query, and you must do so without asking leading questions. (Refer to Chapter 12 for more on physician queries.)

  Electronic medical and health records (which are also being mandated, slowly but surely) will make ICD-10 transition easier. They can be programmed to require greater specificity when documenting a patient record.

Every member of the office staff should be updated as the implementation progresses and provided access to necessary training. Staff members who need training include physicians, nurses, coders, billers, office managers, and any other member of the clerical staff who will be working with the updated or new software system. Expect the coder-in-chief of your office to coordinate the system upgrades and implementation to allow the workflow to continue without interruption or too much disruption.

Don't try to muddle through alone. Most software manufacturers offer training to assist coders with the transition to ICD-10. In addition, most of the clearinghouses, as well as professional organizations like the AAPC and AHIMA, offer training. The Centers for Medicare & Medicaid Services (CMS) also offers online training, webinars, conferences held in various parts of the country, and audio conferences both live and via CDs that you can purchase for self-paced study.

## Helping the physician work on specifics

The ICD-10 transition wheel has many, many cogs, and none is more important than the physician who provides the documentation that gets the coding ball rolling. After all, you can't code anything unless you have a medical record from which to gather information. That's why helping docs understand their role — as ambassadors of detail — in the ICD-10 transition is so very important.

Here are some things you can do to help the physicians get ready:

✔ **Review existing medical records to see how they would meet ICD-10 documentation requirements.** This activity will helps you evaluate whether the level of specificity in the current medical record documentation is sufficient (or lacking) for the ICD-10 requirements.

✔ **Make a list of the kind of documentation that's insufficiently specific (and therefore doesn't meet ICD-10 reporting requirements) and show the physician what steps he needs to take to close the information gap.** Possible documentation lapses include clarification as to whether a condition is acute or chronic, for example — info that's needed to choose the correct code.

In general, documenting a generalized condition such as pneumonia no longer suffices. Physicians need to indicate whether the illness is viral (what virus is suspected or identified) or bacterial (identify the bacterial strain), whether this is the first known infection, and where the infection has settled (in what part of the lung, for example).

# Moving beyond ICD-10

With the huge push toward ICD-10 (despite the U.S.'s delays), no one can blame you for thinking that, after having finally made the transition, you can sit back in the happy glow of having mastered ICD-10 requirements in your billing and coding.

Well, consider that the World Health Organization is expected to have the initial version of ICD-11 ready for public viewing by May 2012 and the final version by 2016. Just like the ICD-10 version, ICD-11 is expected to be structured differently both from a clinical perspective and a technological standpoint.

If history is a predictor, U.S. billers and coders will get comfortable with ICD-10 as other industrialized countries around the world are using ICD-11, again leaving the U.S. behind.

As a coder, always focus on continuing education that not only reinforces current procedures but that also prepares you for the next level. For example, coders who have already achieved ICD-10 certification (there aren't many) are demanding higher salaries from new and current employers. The coders who have been certified to train ICD-10 are even more in demand. A wise coder (and that's you, of course) will always be current on trends and predicted transitions.

# Part V
# Working with Stakeholders

The 5th Wave          By Rich Tennant

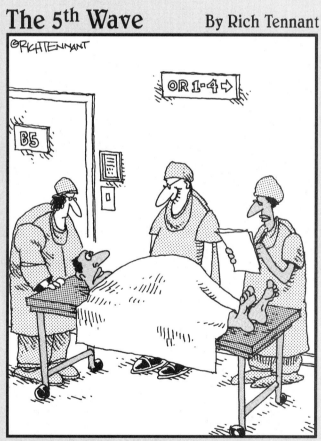

"Included with today's surgery, your PPO insurance plan offers a manicure, pedicure, haircut, and ear wax flush for just $49.95."

## In this part . . .

Time to brush up on your people skills! What? You thought that working as a medical biller and coder would just involve you and your coding software? Well, think again. This gig is all about people. Sure, you'll spend a great deal of time working with codes and software and what seems to be an endless parade of compliance rules and regulations. But you'll also work with people: your clients, your payers, and the patients that come through your office. In this part, I tell you who the stakeholders are and how to do all the tasks your job requires while maintaining your integrity.

# Chapter 16

# Dealing with Commercial Insurance Claims

*Y*ou're going to connect with all sorts of people and organizations in your journey as a medical biller and coder, from individual patients and providers to big, all-encompassing organizations like Medicare. And smack in the middle of all these stakeholders are the Big Boys themselves — the commercial insurance companies. How you work with those insurance companies greatly affects your provider's bottom line. After all, they are the ones writing the checks, so it pays to know how to make the most of your relationship with them. This chapter has the details.

## Meeting Commercial Insurance

As I explain in Chapter 6, most commercial payers, or insurance companies, offer several different levels of coverage to their members, ranging from health maintenance organizations (HMOs) to preferred provider organizations (PPOs) and point-of-service groups (POSs). You'll also run into exclusive provider option plans, high deductible plans, discount plans, and ultra-specific plans that provide only prescription coverage, vision coverage, or other specialized coverage. All of these various flavors of commercial insurance come into play as your claims process.

The commercial insurance world revolves on an axis of variety. From PPO to HMO and in between, a commercial insurance plan exists for just about every situation. Some of these plans are even combinations or iterations of other existing plans. No matter what plans you work with, though, the bottom line is that your provider's bottom line is your ultimate priority. For that reason, one of your top priorities should be to know which commercial insurance products are included in the provider contract, the reimbursement level associated with each product, and the eccentricities of each commercial insurance plan you encounter.

## Big names in commercial insurance

You probably already know the names of some of the most common insurance companies. How can you not? Healthcare and the insurance industry are constantly popping up in the news, and many of them run huge PR campaigns that blanket everything from billboards to your TV. These commercial insurance companies basically underwrite the policies or group plans that the patients and employers pay for. Some of the larger, more well-recognized players in the commercial insurance game are UnitedHealthcare, Aetna, Cigna, and Coventry. These companies are nationwide and offer all types of healthcare plans for their membership.

Another big dog on the commercial insurance block is BlueCross BlueShield (BCBS). This commercial group may, in fact, be the largest of the bunch. The Blue Cross Blue Shield Association has 38 different companies that operate independently yet allow full reciprocity among plans. In other words — and in most cases — if a provider is contracted with a local Blue Cross association, the contract is honored by out-of-state BCBS plans.

This reciprocity makes life a bit easier for BCBS patients who may need care outside of their local zones. Specifically, a provider contracts with the local BCBS company, known as the *local plan*. Some companies that operate in different locations around the country get a plan that's local to the company but underwritten by BCBS affiliates that cover employees who live elsewhere. Claims are submitted to the local BCBS, where they're priced based on the provider's contract. Then they're sent to the sponsoring BCBS company for payment. This way, the patient gets covered, no matter what.

Because commercial insurance companies are the bread and butter of the industry, providers contracted with the major commercial insurance companies have a solid patient base. As such, you can expect to spend a majority of your time working with these payers.

## The benefits of having a contract

The providers for whom you work already know the importance of a strong relationship with commercial insurance payers. In fact, being a contracted provider/member of the commercial insurance company's network offers many benefits: When a provider participates with an insurance company, the provider's name appears on materials and websites that the company produces, which serves as an advertisement of sorts for the individual provider. For physicians who are opening practices, the payer network directs patients to them. Another advantage to contracting with an individual insurance company is that the company defines payment schedules (that is, it clearly outlines the reimbursement amount for each procedure); this information assists the provider in financial planning — and assists you with keeping sane. Just remember: Make nice with the Big Boys, and your provider gets paid. It's a win-win!

## *Working with the major players*

As the coder, you and all members of the office staff who are part of the revenue cycle should be familiar with the provider's commercial payers. Specifically, you need to know the following:

- ✔ **Where the majority of commercial insurance accounts receivable are located.** This info lets you know where the accounts receivable is based.

- ✔ **How much revenue is associated with each payer.** This info lets you know where the accounts receivable (outstanding payments) are to be found.

- ✔ **The eccentricities associated with each payer.** These include things such as timely filing requirements, timely payment obligations, and the other obligations outlined in each payer's contract.

Here's the best bit of advice I can give you when you work with several commercial insurance payers: Because each commercial payer is different, always, always follow the pertinent contract as you move claims through the coding process. The payer contract (which you can read more about in Chapter 11) is the final word on what you can and cannot code, so stick to it like glue.

Although you must bill each carrier as obligated by the individual contract, varying the charge schedule for different payers is unethical. Suppose, for example, that the fee for a certain procedure is $5,000, and most payers have a reimbursement allowance based on the CPT (procedural) code, but one contract pays a percentage of the billed amount. In this situation, changing the fee when you're billing the carrier that pays a percentage of the amount isn't ethical. As a coder, you should not bill carriers different amounts unless a contract that obligates billing according to a specific formula stipulates that you do so.

# Cashing In with Commercial Payers

Commercial insurance pays providers in its own way. Thankfully, that way is not in barter. Rest assured, it's real money. But how you go about getting that cash for your provider can vary, depending on the insurance company. Sometimes, a commercial payer bases how it doles out cash on what Uncle Sam does; more often, procedures are priced based on the amount of work involved by the physician plus a whole host of other factors. In the following sections, I discuss a few of those factors, both standard and rare, beginning with the basics of how reimbursement is determined.

## How reimbursement is determined

Here's a quick breakdown of how the docs get paid. The amount of work associated with each procedure is represented by the RVU, or relative value unit (you read about RVUs in Chapter 13). The Centers for Medicare & Medicaid Services (CMS) assigns an RVU to each CPT code, and the amount is reviewed at least every five years. Medicare fee schedules are based on RVUs. Commercial insurance company payer contracts are often based on either Medicare fee schedules or RVUs; some are based on both (the payment allowance for a particular CPT code may be based on the Medicare fee schedule, for example, while the multiple procedural discount clause is based on RVUs for prioritization).

The other factor that determines reimbursement is the geographical location of the provider. Commercial payers all understand that operating a practice in a major metropolitan area, where the cost of living is higher, takes more money than operating the same kind of practice in a less populated, rural area, where the cost of living is lower. For this reason, actual reimbursement includes the cost of maintaining an office and other overhead expenses, like the malpractice expense associated with particular procedures.

Commercial payment is also based on contract allowances if a contract is in effect on the date of service. When no contract exists to dictate reimbursement, the service provider has the right to demand payment in full for services provided. That's why fees are often based on the same Medicare fee schedule that contracts are based on. Providers usually bill a multiple of the Medicare allowances.

As I note in the section "Working with the major players," regardless of how you compute the billed charges, you should bill every payer the same: If a procedure costs $2,000, then the cost is $2,000 for every claim. Keep in mind, however, that although all insurance companies are billed the same, expectations regarding reimbursement are payer-specific and include things like procedures that may or may not be covered and how long the payer has to send payment.

## Navigating the ins and outs of pricing networks

Here's a point that confuses many people: They think that insurance companies and pricing networks (which are often referred to as "insurance networks" by laypeople) are the same thing. They're not. Commercial insurance companies and pricing networks are two different things. A pricing network is not necessarily the payer of claims; instead, the network prices the claims. The plan administrator or payer issues the payment. Some commercial payers participate in pricing networks rather than do the contracting themselves. In fact, they may participate in several networks simultaneously.

Because pricing networks work on the behalf of commercial payers, you need to know a bit about them. I explain pricing networks in detail in Chapter 6, but in the following sections, I highlight the things you need to keep in mind as you work with them.

### Serving as middlemen

Network pricing companies are essentially the middlemen between the provider and the payer. Like individual insurance company payer contracts, pricing network contracts obligate a significant discount of the provider's fees. Most providers contract with the pricing networks that serve the patients in their geographic area so that they can be in-network with the commercial payers who participate in the pricing network.

Some pricing networks price claims for commercial payers but don't actually have a contract with the service provider. In this case, the provider is not obligated to accept the network's discounted fee and can demand that the unauthorized discount be removed, thus allowing full billed charges. For this reason, the provider must be vigilant about identifying which payers are included in the network when contracting with a network. You can read more about that topic in the section "Avoiding network pitfalls: The silent PPO," coming up shortly.

So that everyone knows what to expect, providers should identify the plans and networks they participate in, and patients (or the patients' payers) should identify the network(s) to which they belong. As the coder (and person who gets to navigate all of this contract madness), you want to stay in close touch with your provider so that you know whenever a contract with a new payer has been entered into so that you can stay on top of the network details.

To know which pricing contract to apply to any particular claim, you must see the patient's insurance card.

### Avoiding network pitfalls: The silent PPO

When contracting with a network, providers must demand that all plans that access the network are identified up-front and that the provider be notified when new payers are added to the network.

The downfall of some network contracts is that, sometimes, payers can get in the network through the back door. That is, these payers are allowed to access the network contract without being identified initially as a network member. This is known as a *silent PPO,* and it's not a good thing for your provider.

Here's how a silent PPO works: Sometimes a PPO network contract contains language that essentially allows the network to enter into a contract with any "individual, organization, firm, or governmental entity" on a case-by-case basis, which means that any payer who is willing to pay the commission can access the PPO contract — and its negotiated discount pricing — *unknown to the provider.* See the problem?

With a silent PPO, a payer can apply a discount rate for services from a healthcare provider without actually having a contract with the provider. This scenario is unfair to providers who sign a contract with the network and its members, which, at the time of signing, did not include the silent PPO. As a result, when the silent PPO pays the discounted rate, it cheats the provider out of a fair payment.

Here are some ways to identify and avoid falling victim to a silent PPO:

✔ **Pay attention to the explanation of benefits (EOB).** You can spot when a payer accesses a silent PPO if you look at the EOB (explained in Chapter 13). If it reflects a PPO discount for a patient who is actually out-of-network, a silent PPO alarm should sound for you.

✔ **Avoid networks that allow reimbursement that is much higher than what other commercial insurance companies allow.** Payers are in business to make money. If a payer is willing to pay more than the going rate, you can bet that it's getting money on the other side — from the organization that is actually responsible for the payment. For example, if a billed service of $1,500 is normally paid $500 but a certain network is willing to pay $750, then that other $250 is coming from somewhere. Chances are, it's coming from the non-network payer who is willing to pay $1,000 to the network rather than $1,500 to the service provider.

✔ **Verify network benefits as part of your provider's normal pre-encounter work.** Either you (or the front office staff) should check the network affiliations on each patient's card.

If you or your provider learns that a network PPO is allowing access to out-of-network payers, then the provider should notify the PPO network that the contract has been violated and terminate the agreement. The provider may also dispute any silent PPO payments in writing with demand for payment in full for services provided.

Being vigilant is the hallmark of a good coder, and that's even more true when you find yourself working with commercial insurance payer networks, whether you patients are in- or out-of-network. Think of yourself as the sheriff of Payertown and keep a watchful eye on shady networks and payers.

## Getting paid in- and out-of-network

One big benefit of working within a network is that the contract usually allows the provider to secure a percentage of billed charges. The payer typically offers a standardized fee structure, and the two parties can (hopefully) reach an agreement that benefits both, which means less work for you and more reliable payments for your provider. Hooray for being in-network!

When a provider is not a participating member of a network, payment can be delayed for a variety of reasons. Often, a payer uses a third-party negotiator to get a discounted reimbursement agreement (you can read about third-party agreements later in this chapter, in the section "Finessing third-party administrators"). Other times, the payer may simply pay a claim based on the reimbursement allowances of other network providers in the area.

If a discount is applied to a claim without a prior agreement, the provider may be able to demand additional payment (refer to the earlier section "Avoiding network pitfalls: The silent PPO" for details). The exception is when the payment is based on the provisions of the patient's individual plan. What this means is that commercial insurance companies offer various levels of coverage, and these plans specify out-of-network benefits and define how much the insurance company pays versus what the patient is responsible for paying.

When a patient is being seen out-of-network, make sure you verify benefits before the encounter. Do the following:

1. **Verify that the patient has out-of-network coverage.**

   Some plans specify an out-of-network payment cap that may be much less than billed charges. The plan then may assign responsibility for the remainder of the balance to the patient. Sometimes this balance is quite large, and most people have difficulty paying it. Occasionally an out-of-network claim processes to allow full-billed charges and then pays according to the plan, usually 60 or 70 percent after the deductible has been met.

2. **Ask what, if any, language in contained in the plan benefit that defines exactly how out-of-network claims are processed.**

3. **If possible, verify what methods may be used to price out-of-network claims, which lets you know how much payment can be expected.**

   The payer representative will always provide the out-of-network deductible and co-insurance responsibility, but that's usually the extent of the information you'll receive. Although getting the payer to divulge the provisions of the plan in question is very difficult, it's worth a try.

Regardless of whether the claim is in- or out-of-network, always treat the payer with respect and give each one equal consideration. The claim should be billed in good faith and be a truthful representation of the work done by the provider.

## Working your way around Workers' Comp carriers

Just when you thought it was safe to code, along comes Workers' Compensation. Workers' Compensation carriers underwrite policies that employers carry to cover treatment for injuries or illness that occur as a result of employment. Processing Workers' Comp claims adds yet another layer to the already teetering tower of things you need to know as a coder.

When you're dealing with Worker's Comp services, keep in mind the following points:

✔ **Workers' Comp claims are normally specific regarding which diagnosis code and body part are authorized for treatment.** In fact, workers may have multiple claims, with a different claim number for each body part.

When verifying a Workers' Compensation claim prior to an encounter, always check the approved diagnosis and body part connected to the claim number.

✔ **Follow-up treatments may be part of the claim.** For this reason, ask for documentation of the history of a particular illness or injury.

Here's an example: A patient who broke her arm had pins put in to reinforce a fracture repair. Now she comes back in complaining of pain because of the hardware. If the fracture was part of a Workers' Comp claim, then removing the hardware is part of the original claim. Similarly, if a patient returns for a hardware removal, and it's scheduled as a Workers' Compensation claim but you see that the original treatment was billed and paid by private insurance, you can contact the Workers' Comp carrier to verify that the claim should have been billed to them. Then you can voluntarily refund the dollars paid to the commercial carrier.

✔ **Sometimes, a Workers' Compensation carrier subrogates a claim with the patient's commercial insurance and simply reimburses the commercial insurance for a claim paid in error.** This action is unfair to the provider because the Workers' Comp carrier benefits from a contracted discount that shouldn't have been used to price the claim. Make sure you catch errors of this nature before any outside negotiation occurs between the carriers.

Subrogation is the process where one insurance company determines that another payer was responsible for claim payment. In this case, the insurance company that paid the claim can demand restitution from the company that was actually responsible. You can read more about subrogation in Chapter 13.

✔ **Some Workers' Comp carriers are part of a PPO network (or several networks).** For your sanity, make sure that your PPO network contracts do not allow silent PPO access (refer to the earlier section "Avoiding network pitfalls: The silent PPO"). Figuring out how to handle Workers' Comp claims is challenging enough; a silent PPO situation only slows the process.

Some states have Workers' Compensation laws that serve as contracts for any provider who offers services under claims filed in that state. This is another factor to consider when negotiating a PPO network contract. Verbiage that states a discount is applied to the fee schedule rather than to the billed charges prevents double discounting.

# Finessing third-party administrators

A third-party administrator (TPA) is an entity hired to handle the administration of another company's insurance plan. The TPA is usually responsible for collecting premiums and issuing reimbursements, which includes paying medical claims.

Companies who use TPAs are required to notify plan participants in writing what the responsibilities of the TPA are. Typically, companies that use TPAs self-insure, which means that they function as insurance companies themselves. As such, they normally join a PPO network as a way to get the advantage of discounted claim pricing while retaining the right to determine deductibles, coinsurance amounts, co-pay obligations, and other plan provisions.

The company plans are funded by payments made by both the employer and participating employees (in the form of premiums). These payments go into a fund that the company owns and that is dedicated to paying claims made against the company's health plan. Here are things to keep in mind about these plans:

- ✔ **They allow employers to customize what the plan covers to best serve the needs of the company's employees.** In some of these plans, injuries or conditions that are common results of work-related duties are excluded from the plan benefit for the employee and delegated as Workers' Compensation claims. For example, a condition such as carpal tunnel syndrome may be identified as a work-related condition, in which case, all carpal tunnel claims are automatically denied upon submission. If, however, the patient is a plan dependent (an individual, such as a spouse or child, who is covered by another person's insurance) rather than an employee, the provider needs to contact the payer and ask that the denial be reconsidered.

- ✔ **The employer or insurance company pays for the TPA's services, not the member directly.** A third-party administrator can only collect payments for plan premiums from plan members.

- ✔ **The payer is responsible for determining the coverage benefit as it applies to each claim.** The TPA only issues the payment. Therefore, if payment is not correct, you need to contact the payer, not the TPA, because the payer is the one who determines whether the claim is payable under the conditions of the patient's insurance plan.

- ✔ **You have to determine where to send the claim.** The payer pays a fee to participate in a network, and the arrangement the payer has with the network determines where you send the claim. Here are the standard options:

- If the network collects fees from both the provider and the payer, you usually submit the claim directly to the network, which prices everything and then requests that the payer present an EOB and a check to the provider.

- If only the payer pays the network, you send the claim to the payer, the payer sends it to the network for pricing, and the network returns the claim to the payer for payment to be issued.

And you, oh lucky coder, get to monitor and follow up on the whole big process, sort of like a big-time TV producer watching all of the magic from a secure location.

# Knowing What's What: Verifying the Patient's Plan and Coverage

Perhaps it goes without saying, but to do your job well, you need to know not only the difference between the types of commercial providers (which the preceding sections in this chapter explain), but also their network affiliations, kind of coverage, and more. Why? Because submitting a claim to the wrong entity delays correct processing. The few minutes it takes to verify benefits and claim submission requirements can save days in accounts receivable and hours of follow-up chasing the claim.

Luckily, gathering the information you need is a fairly straightforward task, as I explain in the next sections.

## Looking at the insurance card

How do you tell what kind of plan — a PPO network, a TPA, or a commercial payer — a patient has? Fortunately, a commercial insurance company that underwrites plans and administers those plans for the membership is usually easy to identify. Just look at the patient's insurance card.

The card provides phone numbers for members and providers to call. By calling the appropriate number, you can get a summary of plan benefits. Most commercial payers also have websites that enrolled providers can use to verify benefits and eligibility.

A company that is self-funded but part of a larger network (or networks) has a benefit and eligibility number on the patient's card, along with the address to which claims are to be sent. It also has the logos for the networks to which it belongs. When you verify these patient benefits, you may need to call both the payer and the network.

A patient is your first line of defense with verifying payer information. Treat each patient with respect and assure him that you're trying to do your job, which is to help his claim get processed in a timely and accurate fashion.

## Contacting the payer and/or network

When you (or the front office staff) call to verify coverage, your first call is probably to the payer, who can verify plan benefits with regard to in-network coverage and out-of-network coverage. The payer can also advise you about any remaining deductibles, coinsurance responsibilities, and applicable co-pays. If the provider participates only in certain levels of the network (say, if the provider is a PPO-provider only), then you want to verify the patient's PPO benefits.

If you have any doubt about coverage, the next step is to contact the network and verify that the payer does actually participate in the network with which the provider has a contract. If the provider is PPO only, verify that the plan is enrolled in the network PPO. If you don't fully verify eligibility and benefits when a network is the pricing intermediary, you can't be certain that the claim will process as expected.

# Chapter 17

# Caring about Medicare

*I*f you haven't spent much time with your uncle lately, prepare yourself because you're going to get to know him very, very well. I'm talking about Uncle Sam, of course, also known as the United States government, also known — for your purposes — as Medicare and Medicaid. These government payers, along with a few others, make up a huge portion of the payers with whom you'll work to secure payment for your provider. Medicare and Medicaid are a big deal because they pay out boatloads of cash to providers each and every day. In addition, these government payers also set the standard for many coding and billing procedures that you use for commercial payers.

Medicare was signed into law by President Lyndon B. Johnson in 1965 as part of the Social Security Act. It was designed to provide healthcare insurance for citizens 65 and over and individuals with certain disabilities. What started as a way to protect the country's most vulnerable populations continues today as one of the country's most widely recognized social programs — and one that you'll work with a lot as a medical biller and coder.

## The Nuts and Bolts of Medicare

At the top of the government heap is the biggest government payer of them all: good old Medicare. Medicare is funded by payroll taxes deducted from every employed American. (You've probably seen the acronym FICA, which stands for Federal Insurance Contributions Act, on your pay stub. This FICA deduction is what helps fund Medicare.)

Everyone who gets a paycheck gets FICA withheld, but you don't see the dividends of that investment until you actually qualify for Medicare. Here's how you can tell whether you (or any patients in your office) fall into that category. Generally those eligible for Medicare are

- Legal U.S. residents who are 65 or older who paid FICA for at least 10 years
- Individuals who are suffering end-stage renal disease who are receiving dialysis treatments or are on a kidney transplant list
- Individuals who are eligible for Social Security Disability Insurance and are suffering from a permanent disability

Medicare has different levels of coverage, referred to as *Parts*. The coverage a patient gets is determined by how that patient paid (or continues to pay) into the plan. Here's a brief overview:

- **Part A** has already been paid for through the patient's payroll taxes. It is primarily considered hospital insurance that covers inpatient care, short-term skilled nursing facility care, some hospice care, and certain home healthcare.
- **Part B** is paid for through deductions, usually from the patient's Social Security dividends. It covers physician services and outpatient services, including outpatient facility fees and other medically necessary services (like physical and occupational therapy) that Part A doesn't cover. Medicare Part B pays 80 percent of covered expenses after patients meet the annual deductible (which is determined each year by Congress).
- **Part C:** Part C, added to the program in 1997, allows individuals who are eligible for Medicare to enroll in Medicare replacement plans offered by private health insurance plans. These plans must meet or exceed Medicare standards and must be approved by Medicare.
- **Part D:** Part D is the new kid on the Medicare block, having been adopted in 2006: It's the drug plan. Part D covers prescription drug coverage. To be eligible for Part D, individuals must be eligible for Part A and Part B. To participate in Part D, a person has to enroll in a prescription drug plan or a Medicare replacement plan that includes drug coverage. These plans are regulated by Medicare, and they don't relieve the patient completely of financial responsibility.

You can read all about these Parts and more in Chapter 6.

# *Working with Medicare Claims*

Think of Medicare like a nice, distant relative who sends you a check for $7 each year for your birthday. It's not flashy, but it's reliable. In other words, Medicare should be your most predictable payer. How so? Well, the fine folks at Medicare provide you with as much information as possible so that you can do your job effectively (and they can do theirs).

Medicare policies and procedures are available on both the Centers for Medicare & Medicaid Services (CMS) website (www.cms.gov), as well as all the local contractor websites. Medicare also reliably follows NCCI edits, and it recognizes modifiers and the payments that link to them. Medicare, for the most part, lets providers know upfront what to expect.

Here's how your provider gets paid with Medicare: Medicare Parts A and B (what's considered "original" Medicare) is administered through regional contractors that accept and process Medicare claims in accordance with Medicare policy. Part B providers are paid per fee schedules, which are available on the your local contractor's website. Fee allowances are based on relative value unit (RVU) equations (I discuss RVUs in Chapter 13).

## Getting Medicare-approved

Before a provider can receive payment for treating a Medicare patient, the provider must apply for Medicare's approval. The registration process to become a Medicare provider takes several weeks to complete. The enrollment forms are available on the CMS website (www.cms.gov), and you can complete most of the enrollment online. To enroll with Medicare, providers must be licensed professionals and have both a National Provider Identification (NPI) number and a tax identification number (TIN). After completing registration, Medicare assigns a Provider Transaction Access Number (PTAN), which allows providers to check claims.

Providers who are not registered cannot submit claims to Medicare, period. As the biller/coder for a provider, you will likely be responsible for leading the effort to fill out all the necessary paperwork to get your provider Medicare-ready.

Registering with Medicare does not automatically mean that a provider is a participating provider. A provider can be registered with Medicare and be what the pros call *non-par* (non-participating). If a patient visits a non-par registered provider, the provider is not obligated to accept fee schedule allowance as payment in full. Instead the provider can charge up to a higher level called a *limiting charge,* and the provider would then need to bill and collect payment from the patient. Medicare reimburses the patient for 80 percent of the fee schedule allowance, but the patient must pay the remaining 20 percent out of his own pocket. Sometimes collecting from patients is difficult, to say the least, so a provider must decide whether to participate with Medicare and receive a lower fee directly from the carrier or risk collecting his fee from the patient at a slightly higher rate.

## Processing Medicare claims

After your provider is good to go as a Medicare provider, you can start processing claims. You submit all claims to the local Medicare contractor, who processes them according to Medicare processing guidelines and policies.

When no national policy applies to a particular service, the decision whether to cover the service may fall to the local Medicare contractor or something called a *fiscal intermediary*, a private insurance company that serves as an agent for the federal government in the administration of Medicare.

The lack of a national policy sometimes happens when a modification has been made with regard to a procedure. Procedural modifications are often the result of advancements in medicine. The development of new tools or equipment that may be used by physicians can result in new procedural codes, for example. Initially, these items are represented by unspecified codes, which are not reimbursable by Medicare. Subsequently, new codes are added to represent these services or items.

Similarly, when a claim is processed incorrectly, the initial appeal process goes through the local contractor, although the process is uniform for all regions.

# LCDs, NCDs, ABNs — OMG! Deciding What Gets Paid

Wouldn't it be nice if, as the coder, you got to make the final call on what gets paid? That certainly would make life easier! But you're not the one writing the checks. Uncle Sam is. For that reason, the government has set up a hierarchy of who gets to make the final decision on some of those tough call situations. In the following sections, I walk you through the more common steps in the decision-making hierarchy and explain how to keep track of them all.

## Going from local to national decision making: LCDs and NCDs

When a contractor or fiscal intermediary makes a ruling as to whether a service or item can be reimbursed, it is known as a *local coverage determination* (LCD). This determination is always based on medical necessity (which you can read more about in Chapter 5).

LCDs apply only to the area served by the contractor who made the decision. Procedural codes that are LCD-dependent are noted as such in the CPT manual. If the provider is planning on submitting a procedural code or HCPCS code that's noted to be subject to an LCD determination, you need to verify the guidelines for the item in question prior to submission.

Sometimes, however, requests are made directly to CMS for a ruling as to whether a service or item may be covered. When CMS makes a decision in response to one of these requests, it's known as a *national coverage determination* (NCD). These rulings specify the Medicare coverage of specific services on a national level. All Medicare contractors are obligated to follow NCDs.

If an item or service is new, or not defined by an NCD, the local contractor is responsible for the decision for coverage. When neither an NCD or LCD exists and it's uncertain whether a service or item will be covered, but the patient desires the treatment or item, the provider must secure an advance beneficiary notice (ABN) prior to the service if he intends to bill the patient. I cover ABNs in the next section.

Both NCDs and LCDs establish policies that are specific to an item or service. They also define the specific diagnosis (illness or injury) for which the item or service is covered. LCDs may vary from region to region. For example, SERVICE 12345 may be covered in Region A to treat diagnosis ABC. But the same service may be covered in Region B only to treat diagnosis XYZ. So when an item or service is in question, always check beforehand (see the later section "Tracking the guidelines: The Medicare Coverage Database"). If a Medicare beneficiary receives an item or service that is not a covered benefit and has not signed an ABN, the provider usually has to absorb the cost.

## Using an advance beneficiary notice (ABN)

As the coder, you're responsible for abstracting reimbursable procedures from the medical record. When the provider performs services or provides items that are not reimbursable and for which there is no LCD, then you can bring the matter to the attention of the office management or the provider to discuss the need for something called an *advance beneficiary notice* (ABN).

The ABN is basically a waiver of liability that providers use when they plan to perform a service that Medicare most likely will determine is not medically necessary. The provider gives the ABN to the patient to sign. After the ABN has been obtained, the provider can hold the Medicare patient liable for the charges. This advanced warning is Medicare's way of insisting that providers inform their patients when Medicare may not reimburse them and alerting the patients to the fact that they will owe the entire amount billed.

## Procedures that are unnecessary... except when they aren't

In certain circumstances, items or services are not covered by Medicare, but in other circumstances, they may be covered. For example, Medicare doesn't cover any cosmetic procedures, but when a normally cosmetic procedure is medically necessary, Medicare may cover it. Consider these examples:

✔ Blepharoplasty is surgery to remove excess tissue from the eyelid and surrounding tissue. Normally, Medicare doesn't cover this procedure. But if the tissue prevents the patient from seeing, Medicare may cover the surgery.

✔ Medicare won't pay to have skin lesions removed (even from the face) just because the patient doesn't like the way the lesion makes him or her look. But if the lesion is painful, impairs vision, or may be malignant, then Medicare covers its removal.

These "sometime they're covered; sometimes they're not" scenarios are not limited solely to Medicare. You can also find examples in private insurance plans. The need for verification of coverage extends to all healthcare providers. The provider is the professional and is in the best position to be aware of medical necessity and national or local coverage determinations.

Currently, providers can customize their own ABN forms as long as the forms contain the required language. Generally, the ABN must be easy to read; use a large font size; and identify the provider, the patient, the service or item in question, and the reason that payment is expected to be denied. In addition, the patient must sign the ABN every time the service or item is provided. (You can't have patients sign a blanket form that obligates them to pay for a service not deemed necessary by Medicare.) CMS requirements regarding correct notifications are available on the CMS website (www.cms.gov).

## *Tracking the guidelines: The Medicare Coverage Database*

Making coverage decisions is a big deal, and the government doesn't take these decisions lightly. The Social Security Act grants Medicare contractors and fiscal intermediaries the authority to make these decisions, which must follow NCD guidelines. In addition, the decision is always in writing.

Thankfully, you can keep track of all these decisions and determinations so that you can use them for future reference. The CMS maintains a Medicare Coverage Database that contains all NCDs and LCDs. Medicare updates this database regularly to keep it as current as possible.

The guidelines that the contractors must follow when making coverage decisions are outlined in the *Medicare Program Integrity Manual.* This manual is part of the Internet Only Manual, which you can find through the CMS website (www.cms.gov) or the Medicare website (www.medicare.gov).

# Working with Medicare Contractors

When you think of Medicare, you probably (or will soon) immediately think of the umbrella organization, the Centers for Medicare & Medicaid Services (CMS). Who you *should* be thinking about are the local Medicare contractors or fiscal intermediaries, because these are the people providers deal directly with.

## Submitting your claims

You submit your claims to the local carrier, who processes them. Each carrier is required to follow Medicare processing guidelines, which help contractors provide the same Medicare level of service to all providers. Each Medicare contractor must do the following:

- ✔ Accept electronic claim submissions

- ✔ Maintain an interactive voice response (IVR) provider phone line

- ✔ Follow the same timely filing requirements set by Medicare

- ✔ Make payment according to Medicare fee schedules and timely payment rules

- ✔ Operate the same way when it comes to the Health Insurance Portability and Accountability Act (HIPAA) communications and observe all HIPAA regulations

Regardless of which contractor you call, you can always expect the process to follow these steps:

1. At the contract's request, you supply the provider's PTAN (provider transaction access number), the provider's NPI (national provider identification number), and the last five digits of the TIN (tax identification number).

   For more information on these numbers, refer to the earlier section "Getting Medicare-approved."

2. You will be asked for the patient's Medicare number, name, and date of birth before any privileged information will be shared.

3. You may then make claim or member-specific inquiries.

By following the same protocols for every single phone call, the contractors allow Medicare to operate with more expedience and efficiency for the large number of claims that are submitted daily.

Regardless of which government program you're dealing with, you work with a regional, or possibly a local, company. Each of these administrators has its own contact information (phone number, electronic payer identification number, and physical address).

## Getting along with your Medicare rep

Each Medicare contractor has provider representatives available for assistance when you're not sure what is wrong with a submitted claim, but these representatives can't advise you how to code or how to bill. They can only direct you to the correct resources that will assist in getting your claim paid.

When calling Medicare, make sure you have the following info handy:

- ✔ The PTAN, the number assigned by Medicare to the individual provider

- ✔ The provider's NPI, the 10 digit provider number that CMS issues

- ✔ The last five digits of the provider's TIN, which is similar to an individual's Social Security number

- ✔ The patient's Medicare number

- ✔ The patient's name and date of birth

- ✔ The date of service and billed amount of the claim in question

# Working with Medicare Part C Plans

As I mention previously, in addition to the Medicare contractors, commercial insurance companies also sponsor Medicare-approved plans. These plans are referred to as Medicare Part C plans, and they sometimes pay differently than standard Medicare plans.

## Paying attention to plan differences

Standard Medicare pays 80 percent of the allowed amount after the patient meets the annual deductible. The other 20 percent is the responsibility of the patient, who can enroll in a Medicare-approved supplemental plan to cover the other 20 percent.

Patients who have chosen a replacement Medicare plan, however, must follow the provisions of that policy. Many of these plans cover 100 percent of the allowed amount after a deductible and/or copay has been met. If your provider is contracted with the parent company that sponsors the replacement plan, the contract dictates how much the claim pays (within the plan provisions).

Your front office needs to know the difference between a commercial insurance plan and a Medicare Part C replacement plan sponsored by the same commercial payer because the distinctions between the two can impact which codes you use. If the provider has a specific Part C contract with the carrier, you follow the carrier's claim process. If the provider doesn't have a specific Part C contract with the carrier, you follow the claim process specified by Medicare's reimbursement policy. The differences between these policies determine which codes you submit.

## *Turning to Uncle Sam for a helping hand*

If the provider has a disagreement with a commercial Medicare payer, you must follow the dispute process defined by that company's policy for the original level-one reconsideration request. Higher level appeals, however, follow the dispute process defined by Medicare. (Head to Chapter 14 for detailed information on requests for reconsideration.)

When a dispute with a private Medicare plan fails to get resolved through the sponsoring company's appeals process, the provider (or beneficiary) may request a review by the Part C independent Review Entity.

Each Medicare Part C sponsoring company must give the provider information regarding which organization to contact if the provider feels that the appeal should be elevated to the next level. This information must be included with the response to the initial request for reconsideration.

If you work in a small office or for a larger company with a focus on accounts receivable follow up, expect this appeals process to be a daily part of your job. The request for reconsideration is the initial level of appeal, when a provider feels that the claim has not processed correctly. If the reconsideration is denied, then the second-level appeal goes through an independent review. If the provider is still unsatisfied with the outcome of the request, the same appeals process that standard Medicare requests follow applies. I discuss this process in Chapter 14.

## *Verifying Coverage and Plan Requirements*

Medicare and Medicaid plans must follow federal guidelines, but each policy can have other specified requirements, as well. These requirements are similar to those of most HMO plans, restricting patients to contracted providers, for example, or requiring prior authorization for treatment beyond the primary care provider services.

Although both Medicare and Medicaid fall under the jurisdiction of the U.S. Department of Health & Human Services, there is no national Medicaid program. Instead, each state voluntarily sponsors its own program, often through commercial carriers. Medicaid must work within the guidelines (such as meeting eligibility requirements for members), but beyond that, each state can do its own thing. Medicare, on the other hand, is a national program, and it must be administered as dictated by CMS.

## Checking in on plan specifics

You absolutely must know the specific coverage requirements for the plans that sponsor your patients. Prior to any patient encounter, look on each patient's insurance card for the provider inquiry phone number to call to verify benefits and payer specific policies.

### Checking the insurance card or payer website

Most of these plans assign responsibility for denied services to the provider. Patients who qualify for Medicaid assistance (the insurance program designed for the poor), for example, are unlikely to personally have the resources to pay out of pocket for denied medical services. Even if the payer denies coverage and indicates that the patient is responsible for the charges, the provider still isn't going to get paid if the patient doesn't have the money.

Medicaid policies that are sponsored by private payers are sometimes difficult to locate. Because each state is responsible for Medicaid program administration and the states often rely on commercial carriers to facilitate these programs, you need to be familiar with these payer guidelines. Ideally, the payer is one that maintains a website that lets providers and the coders view the payer policies.

### Looking in the plan's provider contract

In some cases, commercial payers who underwrite Medicaid plans include these plans with their other commercial products in the provider contracts. Having this info in the contract can be beneficial to providers, but you need to make sure that the payer intended for all products to be included. Most payer contracts, however, clearly identify which products are included; any product not listed is excluded.

Make sure you don't assume, just because your provider has a contract with Payer ABC, that Payer ABC's Medicaid plan has the same requirements as its standard plan. Don't assume, for example that the provider can see Medicaid patients without the required referral or prior authorization. Similarly, don't assume that, just because a referral or authorization was not necessary six months ago, it's not needed next week.

When verifying coverage for Medicaid patients, make sure you verify all possible scenarios that may occur in the course of the patient's treatment plan. If a particular procedure is a possibility, call the carrier, give the representative the corresponding code to make sure that that service is covered, and secure any necessary authorization.

## *Obtaining referrals and prior authorizations*

As I mention previously, the provider is responsible for securing the necessary referrals and authorizations.

Make sure you're familiar with the difference between a referral and prior authorization. A *referral* is issued by the primary care physician, who sends the patient to another healthcare provider for treatment or tests. A *prior authorization* is issued by the payer, giving the provider the go-ahead to perform the necessary service.

Here are some things to keep in mind about referrals and prior authorization for Medicare and Medicaid services:

- ✔ **Standard Medicare does not require referrals or prior authorization for procedures that meet medical necessity and do not require any type of NCD or LCD.** Fortunately, these represent the majority of treatment options.

- ✔ **A Medicare HMO or Medicaid patient who needs prior authorization before being treated by a specialist or to receive services provided by a facility needs a referral or authorization for *each* provider and possibly for each visit.**

    If you get an authorization over the phone, always make note of the name of the representative with whom you spoke, along with the date and time of the call. If authorization was obtained via a payer web portal, print the screen for proof, just in case you need it later.

- ✔ **Some authorizations cover a period of time and/or a specified number of treatments or visits.** Consider this example: A Medicaid or Medicare HMO patient may come to the primary care physician with a broken arm. The physician will probably authorize the patient to see an orthopedic surgeon for fracture care. The referral may authorize the specialist to diagnosis and treat the patient for up to three visits over a two-month period of time. If the specialist determines that the patient needs surgery, another referral or authorization is needed: The surgeon needs two things: authorization to perform surgery and a referral or authorization to treat the patient (perform the surgery) in the specified facility.

✔ **Authorizations normally are active over a specific date range and may expire if not used during that time.** If the authorization date has passed, you need to contact the payer again and request another authorization.

✔ **The initial referral or authorization doesn't cover additional services.** In my earlier example of the patient with the broken arm, if the services of a physical or occupational therapist are needed, another referral is necessary.

✔ **Obtaining prior authorization is still not a guarantee of payment.** The submitted claim must still be 1) supported by medical necessity, 2) filed within the timely filing requirements, and 3) filed by the provider mentioned in the referral or authorization.

## Oops! Getting referrals and authorizations after the fact

Somebody has to do the paperwork for referrals or prior authorizations, and that somebody is unlikely to be the physician. So whose job is it? Everybody's. The scheduler, the coder, and the biller should all know when a referral or prior authorization is needed. Of course, by the time the case reaches you, the biller/coder, the encounter has already taken place. So what do you do if the necessary referral or authorization wasn't secured before the fact? You play nice.

If you haven't sent the claim yet, it may not be too late to call the payer and secure the necessary referral or authorization. Or you may be able to contact the primary care physician and explain the situation. Often she will issue the necessary number or form that allows the claim to be submitted within the provision of the patient's plan.

If the need for referral or prior authorization goes unnoticed until after the claim has been denied, the job falls to the person responsible for accounts receivable follow up to try to get the retroactive authorization or referral. Sometimes you can obtain this by submitting an appeal along with the medical records to support medical necessity.

Getting hostile with the payer if the claim has been denied because your office didn't do the necessary work up front doesn't benefit anyone. Instead, explain that a miscommunication occurred and that you're sorry for the confusion; then very nicely ask, "What can I do to straighten this out and get the claim paid?" Afterward, to avoid a recurrence, use the denial as a teachable moment for other members of the staff. You also may want to post a list of known payers who require prior authorizations or referrals for services performed in your office.

# Chapter 18

# Client Relations and Coding Ethics: Being an Advocate for Your Employer

- - - - - - - - - - - - - - - - - - - - - - - - - - - - - - - - - - - - - - - - - - - -

## In This Chapter

▶ Communicating effectively — and diplomatically — with payers, patients, and colleagues

▶ Adhering to accepted coding practices in all situations

▶ Protecting yourself against charges of fraud

- - - - - - - - - - - - - - - - - - - - - - - - - - - - - - - - - - - - - - - - - - - -

*T*he medical billing and coding job market offers so many kinds of opportunities that you may feel like you're at a job buffet! Just think of it: You can work in a larger office for a hospital. Or maybe you can set up shop with a billing company that specializes in specific provider types like physician practice management companies, ambulatory surgery center management companies, anesthesia practice management companies, or numerous other specialty services. Maybe you want to focus on one client and work for a physician where you are not only in charge of coding but also responsible for accounts receivable follow up.

Whatever position you find, your fiduciary responsibility is always to your employer. You should always have the best interest of your employer in mind when dealing with payers and patients alike. You are the first and last line of defense when it comes to protecting your client's interests. The best way to protect your client's interests is to comport yourself professionally and follow accepted coding practices. This chapter has the details.

# Playing the Part of the Professional Medical Biller/Coder

To secure timely payment for the provider (that is, your employer or client), you'll find yourself working and communicating with many different people. As a representative of the office, being friendly and approachable to patients and payers alike is fine. After all, the professional demeanor you exhibit toward patients, fellow office staff, your superiors, and the payers with whom you work goes a long way in helping you establish your role as advocate-in-chief. But you must respect professional boundaries and behave in a professional way at all times.

Whether you are discussing missing patient intake information with the front office staff or making your case to a payer representative after being on hold for an hour, you must temper your frustrations with some level of kindness and understanding. Claims processing is business, and you've got to view it and communicate about it objectively, especially when you're doing the detective work of following up on unpaid claims. No matter who you're dealing with — your friends in the front office or your new best buddy George from the Medicare help line — stay focused on the facts. Leave your emotions at the door and stick to what's on the paper or computer screen.

In the following sections, I tell you how to keep the your employer/client at the top of your priority list as you interact with patients, payers, and others.

## Dealing with patients

Although you'll spend the lion's share of your time cozied up to your coding books and software, you occasionally need to interface with patients. In these interactions, your diplomacy chops come in handy. Navigating the sometimes choppy waters of patient relations isn't always easy, especially when the patient with whom you're working may be visibly emotional.

In this kind of situation — or in any situation involving a patient — your best bet is to be courteous, maintain your professional demeanor, and focus on the facts. In the following sections, I explain how to handle some of the more challenging interactions you may have with patients.

Patients are the physician's clients (not yours), so always treat them with respect and empathy. Without patients, healthcare providers would have no revenue, and if they don't get paid, you don't get paid.

### When the patient can't pay the bill

In a way, patients are payers of sorts because, in many cases, they're responsible for at least some portion of the bill you code. For example, a patient may be responsible for a 20 percent co-insurance, meaning she has to pay 20 percent of what you code and bill. (Chapter 6 goes into more detail on insurance plans and the kinds of patient contributions that are commonly expected.)

In a small office setting, you may be the same person who receives a call from the patient who can't pay her bill, and these issues can be very difficult to address. In this situation, remain professional but be sympathetic to the patient's dilemma. Here are some suggestions:

- ✔ **Follow your employer's rules about contacting patients.** Providers let you know when contacting a patient is okay and what method they prefer for this communication.

- ✔ **Identify yourself upfront.** When you call patients, always let them know that you are with Dr. Smith's billing office or the billing office at Smith's Clinic.

- ✔ **Be a listener, not a talker.** You don't need to impart too much information about the inner workings of your client or employer's office to a patient, if any at all. For example, providers don't necessarily want their patients to know when the billing company or representative (you) is off site.

- ✔ **Explain any available payment plan options.** If your office accepts credit cards, installment payments, or financing options, explain those to the patient.

### When the patient doesn't understand how his insurance works

Patients with whom you interact may not fully understand how insurance works, so you may be called upon to explain some insurance basics. These situation often arises when the insurance company sends a payment to the patient instead of the provider by mistake, when a patient receives an explanation of benefits (EOB) statement he doesn't understand, or when the patient receives a bill from the provider that he wasn't expecting.

Many such situations arise when patients are out-of-network and, as a result, are often responsible for a large portion of the bill themselves. In these situations, the following suggestions can help you resolve the issue:

- ✔ **Before making any calls, make sure you know what the provider's policy is regarding out-of-network patients.** If the provider is knowingly treating patients outside of the network, a policy should be in place to address how these claims will be handled.

- ✔ **If the patient receives a check from the insurance company by mistake, it may be your responsibility to call the patient and explain that they need to surrender the check to the provider.** An alternative is to inform the patient of the situation and then bill them for the full charges, explaining that they can use the insurance check to pay the bill. Unfortunately, some patients refuse to surrender the check. In that case, collection agencies get involved or lawsuits are filed.

✔ **Inform patients of payment plan options.** When additional payment is expected of the patient, explain any payment plans that are available, including credit cards or financing options accepted by the provider.

✔ **Always be cordial, even when patients may get angry and direct their anger toward you.** Don't allow yourself to be drawn into an argument. Try to remember that the patient's frustration isn't personal. Keep your comments friendly and professional, and you'll do right by your employer or client.

## Dealing with payers

Your primary goal when interacting with payers is simple: Make sure payers show your client the money! Ideally, your billing software and clearinghouse will keep you apprised of the status of claims (where they are and when they were received) through reports they can generate. The clearinghouse (the agency that relays the claim from the provider to the payer) also generates a batch report that identifies the claims transmitted in each batch. As a result, you should know where every claim is in the process.

Occasionally, however, a claim doesn't process. In that case, you need to talk to a real, live human being to find out why. When calling a payer to follow up on a claim, you are the voice of the healthcare provider, so always act in a professional manner. Remember, being nice gets you better service.

Make note of the representative's first name (and the first initial of her last name) when you call to follow up on a claim, and then use her first name as you talk. People like to hear their own names, so repeat the representative's name back to her. After the rep says, "My name is Sue," you can introduce yourself with, "Hi, Sue. This is John from Provider Smith's office. How are you doing today?" Keep the tone friendly rather than confrontational (at least in the beginning). It doesn't hurt to note the phone number and time of your call either. That way, during subsequent calls, you can use this info to prove that you spoke to someone in the payer's office; this info comes in especially handy if the payer's system doesn't have a record of your call.

### Remaining patient

Normally, the payer representative is required to get three pieces of identification for both the provider and the patient. In most cases, the representative asks you for the provider's name and specific information such as Tax Identification Number (TIN) or National Provider's Identification (NPI) Number. You also need to provide patient name, member identification number, and date of birth. Only after providing this information can the provider representative discuss the specific claim information with you.

## Following your client's lead

You are the voice of the service provider. The best way to know how to act as you advocate for your provider is to mirror the level of professionalism the employer/client sets forth.

Mirroring your client's level of professionalism is especially important when you work in a billing or practice management company. Physicians and other providers are always cautious when entrusting a third-party (your company) to handle their revenue, which is the life blood of the practice. For this reason, you must always remain professional.

Expect your employer or client to define the parameters of your duties as office representative extraordinaire and to define their expectations. If you need additional information prior to submitting a claim, the provider tells you how to ask for it. If your employer/ client wants to be kept apprised of the status of various payments, he or she will let you know what level of daily reporting is required of you. Bottom line: You can start the relationship off right by inquiring about employee-client relationships and expectations. So keep those lines of communication open and let your employer/client lead the way.

Asks for this information isn't a stall tactic on the part of the payer representative. It's required by the Health Insurance Portability and Accountability Act (HIPAA). HIPAA guarantees that a patient's privacy is protected, and only those with a need to know are privy to this protected information.

### Getting the resolution you want

Only after getting through the initial step (proving you have a need to know the patient's confidential information) are you able to inquire about the specific claim in question. Here are some pointers:

- ✔ **If the person with whom you are speaking is unable to assist with your inquiry, ask to be transferred.** When you are transferred to a supervisor, don't cast blame. Simply describe the issue and the reason you feel that the other person was not providing the resolution you need. Let the supervisor know that you have every confidence that he or she can resolve the issue.

- ✔ **If you are still unable to resolve the issue, submit a written request and identify the issue in addition to your expectations.** Make sure you also define the contractual obligation that supports your position. After you submit this written request, follow up with a call to make sure that the request was received and forwarded to the correct department for appropriate action.

- ✔ **Don't threaten or accuse.** Instead, stand behind the claim in question and your expectations as defined by any contract or state laws with regard to claim processing and payment. You don't gain anything by accusing the provider relations representative of failing to process a claim. Instead, ask the representative to help you identify the reason(s) the claim processed incorrectly or was rejected. Make that person your ally, not your adversary.

Any information the representative gives you on the call is *not* a guarantee of payment (in fact, early in your conversation, the representative should tell you that directly). As always, payment depends on the benefits outlined in the patient's individual plan.

## *Providing positive feedback to colleagues*

Part of being a professional is being able to provide positive feedback to co-workers. Let's face it: Office politics are often (okay, always) at play, so getting along with your co-workers is important. From the receptionist at the front desk to the intake nurse, you have multiple opportunities to keep things positive around the office (even if someone's driving you nuts).

The success of your job as a biller/coder depends largely on the accuracy of the information gleaned when each patient checks in. Here are some tips on how to get (or continue to get) the info you need from the front desk:

- ✔ Make sure that the people at the front desk who are facilitating this process understand its importance and let them know how much you appreciate the effort they put into getting cooperation from the patients.

- ✔ If necessary information is often missing or incorrect, examine the form and see whether you can identify a particular area that makes gathering the necessary information difficult. Discuss the issue with the office manager and diplomatically remind the staff that mistakes on the front end of the claim delay payment.

- ✔ If the office uses electronic medical records that employ electronic patient registration, make sure that the necessary information is programmed to the required field.

Most offices that use electronic medical records are contracted with or have their own software support (the Information Technology department). Work with the IT department to make sure that the necessary information is entered.

When discussing deficiencies in an office process or a co-worker's performance, try to use constructive suggestions. The following examples illustrate how to phrase feedback in a positive way. Notice how each identifies the issue and opens the door to a possible solution without accusation or blame:

- ✔ "Do you think that we need to revise the demographic form since we're not always capturing the necessary information up front?"

- ✔ "Do we have a contact at XYZ insurance that we (or I) can reach out to for assistance with this issue?"

- ✔ "I've identified a pattern that shows we're not differentiating between the AEIOU insurance plans when we enter them into the billing software.

> Please make sure to check the address on the each patient's insurance card when entering demographic and billing information."

✔ "Dr. Smith usually does not dictate until being reminded. Can we set up a remote dictation system to make it easier for him?"

✔ "It would make claim submission faster if we had the necessary invoices without requesting them. Can we set up a process to have the invoices copied to the billing office upon receipt?"

✔ "We can't submit claims that are waiting for pathology reports. Is there a way for us to access these reports directly through the lab?"

✔ "If Joe needs help with payer matching, I'd be happy to do it with him" (as opposed to telling Joe you will do it yourself).

✔ "Thanks!" The most important sentence of all.

# Protecting Yourself and Your Integrity

Whether you realize it or not, your position as the person who codes every patient interaction and procedure makes you the most trusted person in the office. Clients and employers trust you not only with their patients' personal and private information, but they also trust you to code accurately, fairly, and legally. To be worthy of this trust, you must maintain your integrity as a medical biller/coder.

From time to time, however, you may find yourself faced with a client, patient, fellow employee, or payer representative who asks you to ignore your own professional standards. In these cases, your integrity must take priority over getting your client paid. By protecting your professional integrity and coding in a way that upholds professional coding standards, you can rest assured that you are doing the best job you can.

## Surviving a sticky situation

When you become a certified coder and biller, you receive instruction in correct coding and claim submission procedures and rules. From that point on and throughout your coding career, you're responsible for observing and promoting those rules.

"But, I have a boss!" you say. Yep, you sure do — probably a coding manager, an office manager, or perhaps the healthcare provider. This person may sign your paychecks, but the onus for correct coding is on *you,* especially when your boss is unaware of or unconcerned about correct coding rules. Even some managers, despite being aware of coding rules, may ignore them. In the following sections, I offer advice on how to deal with both situations.

### Superiors asking you to fudge the coding

Having an office manager challenge the coding of claims when reimbursement is low isn't uncommon, and it puts you in a tough situation. For example, some office managers may want you to use modifiers as a tool to increase reimbursement rather than a tool to increase specificity when reporting services (Chapter 12 covers modifiers).

In cases where a superior wants you to fudge the coding, rely on your coding books for backup. The NCCI edits are a good place to start. If you stick to your correct coding guidelines, you have the facts you need to make coding decisions that maintain your professional integrity.

### Physicians asking you to submit codes the record doesn't support

Some physicians may want to submit procedural codes that the record doesn't support. In this case, you may need to review the code description with the physician and ask for clarification as to why he feels the code is justified. You may discover that he failed to fully document the procedure that was performed.

If, however, you are certain that you correctly abstracted the codes from the record, you can request an independent audit, in which another coder reviews the record and notes which codes he feels are supported by the documentation. If the audit supports your position, you've secured the necessary documentation and you can submit the claim as you coded it originally. If the audit indicates that you are under-billing the claims, you must be willing to alter the way you code. The good news here is that you get the opportunity to make the record right — and you now know how to code more accurately in the future.

If you find yourself in an office that demands coding that is contrary to correct coding standards, despite the results of an independent audit, then it's time to find another job. You should always code and bill ethically. If the employer's business philosophy contradicts those ethics and your integrity, then leave. Acquiescing to unethical standards can get you into big trouble. When (or if) your employer is subject to a request for payment refund, an audit, or accusations of fraudulent billing, not only will those events not look good on your resume; the possibility exists that you will be considered an accomplice.

### Coding resources you can use as support

When you're asked to do something unethical or contrary to accepting coding practices, base your discussions on the guidelines of coding ethics. Resources are available to support correct coding positions and help you know what to say when. These resources include the following:

✔ ***The Coding Edge:*** The monthly publication of the AAPC, this magazine is sent to all AAPC members, and back issues are available on the organization's website (www.aapc.com).

- ✔ *CPT Assistant:* This is an official guide for interpretation of CPT by the American Medical Association and available by subscription.

- ✔ **The Coding Institute:** The Institute offers specialty newsletters that require subscriptions but keep readers abreast of coding developments. Find them at `www.codinginstitute.com`.

- ✔ *Journal of AHIMA:* This journal is available through the AHIMA website (`www.ahima.org`). AHIMA membership also entitles members to access the organization's newsletters.

- ✔ **Medicare and Medicare contractor websites:** You can find volumes of current coding information here.

- ✔ *The Coder's Desk Reference* **(Ingenix/Optum):** This coding book contains detailed descriptions of each CPT code. Ingenix also publishes coding companion books for various specialties that provide more in-depth descriptions of the procedures.

- ✔ **Coding software programs:** Look for those that offer access to expert resources for coding questions or challenging coding scenarios.

- ✔ **The AAPC member forum:** Through this forum, members can post questions to be answered by other members. This information is only as good as the member who provides the answers, though, so use with care. Consider asking the forum participants to cite their official references.

- ✔ *Coder's Pink Sheet,* **by DecisionHealth:** A favorite publication written by many seasoned coders, these newsletters are specific to various specialties. You can purchase a subscription through `www.decisionhealth.com`.

When involved in any type of coding controversy or any interaction that involves a specific claim or account, keep your cool and document all conversations in the record, whether conversations are with payer representatives or patients. As long as you stay positive and professional, the record will reflect that you truly have your client's best interests at heart.

## Documenting your day

A great way to keep all of your coding activities on the up-and-up is to spend some time each day writing down (or typing up) what you work on each day. I like to keep a time log for each project, making special note of any claims that have trouble getting through the claims process.

Not only does such a record keep you up-to-date on deadlines and how things are going with your claims, but it also provides a history should anyone question why certain decisions were made. In your documentation, record any special circumstances that affect a claim, such as the following:

- ✔ The date on which you must submit a corrected claim

- ✔ When a patient calls to make special payment arrangements

✔ Whether a claim was initially rejected and what action was taken

✔ If a claim paid incorrectly, the date the payment was received and the reason it was incorrect

✔ Any action taken as a result of incorrect claims processing, calls, letters, and so on

✔ All circumstances concerning a medical record and the reason the services were necessary (medical necessity)

✔ The patient's consent to services and agreement to be responsible for payment

✔ The date a payment was received and from whom

✔ The date the claim was submitted to the secondary payer and any communication that resulted from that submission

With all claim documentation, make sure that you include the names of the people you spoke to, the date and time that the conversation took place (most software records this automatically), and all details of the conversation.

## Mum's the word: Keeping patient info private

Earning and keeping patient trust starts the moment you sign on for your new billing and coding job. Most healthcare providers require employees and vendors to sign confidentiality agreements. These agreements serve as your acknowledgment that you will keep any patient information confidential.

Keeping patient info confidential isn't just the right thing to do; it's the law as outlined by HIPAA. So when you sign your confidentiality agreement, be sure you mean it. Patient confidentiality is serious business, and violating this confidence may result in a fine or, in serious circumstances, imprisonment. For more information on HIPAA, refer to Chapter 4.

### Steps you can take to protect confidentiality within the office

Patients trust the provider and the provider's staff to protect their personal information. Providers ask for patient Social Security numbers, birth dates, addresses, and other information that opens the door for identity theft. A lot is at stake for your patients when they release this highly personal information to you, and you owe it to them, to the provider, and to yourself to treat it with the utmost care.

# HIPAA and criminal liability

In June 2005, the United States Justice Department issued a clarification regarding who can be held criminally liable under HIPAA. They are the big boys of healthcare: health plans, healthcare clearinghouses, healthcare providers who transmit claims in electronic form, and Medicare prescription drug card sponsors. Individuals such as directors, employees, or officers of the covered entity may also be directly criminally liable.

Any of these entities and individuals who disclose protected health information may face a fine of up to $50,000 and up to one year in prison. Offenses committed under false pretenses can result in fines of up to $100,000 and five years of prison. Offenses that involve intention to sell or use individually identifiable health information for personal gain, commercial advantage, or malice can result in fines of $250,000 and 10 years of prison.

Protecting the patient's personal information begins in the reception area or waiting room. Gone are the days when the nurse or other employee would call a patient by first *and* last name (it gives away a patient's identity to everyone in the waiting room), or when the admitting personnel would ask the patient to explain the reason for the visit in front of other patients (no one wants fellow patients to find out about that unfortunately placed rash).

Today, because of HIPAA, providers have taken great steps to protect patient identity and privacy: Patient records are kept in locked files out of the view of the public. Patient registration information is kept in computers that are password protected and that timeout within a few minutes of inactivity. Passwords for clearinghouse access, software access, and insurance website access must be changed at specified intervals. All employees must have their own usernames and passwords, and sharing their access information with others is a HIPAA violation. These are just a few of the changes.

You can help keep your client's circle of trust intact by working with fellow office colleagues to stay abreast of HIPAA rules and regulations. You can also offer to be the office HIPAA liaison with outside entities, checking in from time to time to find out about their efforts to maintain patient privacy and following up with your client or employer if you suspect any discrepancies.

## Protecting confidentiality when working with others

You're not the only person who has access to a patient's personal information. The healthcare provider obtains permission from the patient to share this personal information with other stakeholders as necessary to receive reimbursement for the services provided. These other stakeholders include the insurance company (which needs to know the reason treatment was provided) and the clearinghouse (which is privy to the patient's personal health information during transmission of the claim). Both clearinghouses and payers must follow the same privacy standards mandated by HIPAA.

## Keeping yourself honest: What to do when you make a mistake

As a biller and coder, you must be self-reliant, because you perform most of your daily office functions independently of others. The same is true of maintaining your ethical standards. You need to police yourself. After all, your job and reputation is on the line if something goes wrong in the coding and claims process, and claims aren't being paid in a timely fashion.

Your first charge is to make sure that you're submitting the claims correctly (refer to Chapters 11 through 13). Then follow them up and, if the claims aren't being paid, identify the reason for the delay and try to have the issue corrected (Chapter 14). Easier said than done, especially when the mistake that delays payment is yours.

Just keep in mind that you're human, and you'll make mistakes. By admitting that you screwed up a claim, you're not only keeping yourself honest, but you're also helping the issue get resolved faster. (Think of the time you'd waste — or the trouble you'd be in — trying to cover up your mistake or deflect blame).

# Getting the Most Bang for Your Client's Buck — Honestly

Your job as a biller/coder is, in plain terms, to get the provider paid for services rendered. Part of that payment comes from the payers, whether they're commercial (health insurance) or governmental (Medicare, Medicaid, and others). The other part of payment often comes from the patients themselves.

## Collecting payments from patients

Yes, your most important job is to fully abstract all billable services and supporting medical necessity from the physician's documentation. But the other part of your job is to follow provider-payer contracts that stipulate that the provider is obligated to collect patient balances. Failure to do so may result in the contracts being canceled.

## Accounts receivable: Your secret ethical weapon

When patients have trouble meeting their financial responsibilities or physicians fail to document, you may be asked to let payments slide or to go ahead and code an encounter that has no documentation. Fortunately, you have a secret weapon you can rely on to drive home the point that fudging just won't work: accounts receivable (AR).

Outstanding revenue needs to be collected (no one knows that better than your boss) before it can be used. Allowing patients to make installment payments is an option, but it increases the AR line on the balance sheet, and the provider can't invest money that hasn't been received, nor can he make payroll until the money is in the bank. The way to avoid this problem is to encourage the provider to collect all known deductibles, anticipated co-insurance amounts, and copayments before the patient encounter and to make patients aware of this practice prior to the date of service. That way, they're prepared to make payment when they arrive."

On the other end of your process is the provider who fails to document. Sure, he may see 75 patients a day with an average of $100 payment per encounter, but if he doesn't dictate until he's faced with the threat of privilege revocation, he can't get the money he obviously wants. Providers like this need to be reminded that they can't get paid until the claim is submitted, and the claim can't be submitted without the documentation. If pressured to fudge your coding process, remind such docs that you won't be able to pursue unpaid claims in AR without the proper provider documentation anyway, so getting paid won't even be an option. That tends to get their pens moving!

 The contract defines the conditions for submitting claims, the procedures to be submitted for payment and the medical necessity that supports the procedures, and reimbursement obligations of both the payer and the patient. When you try to collect payment from patients, you must follow the same principles of honesty and integrity that you follow when you code.

When you follow up on outstanding patient payments, be sure to do the following:

- ✔ **Treat all patients the same, regardless of what kind of insurance they have.** Most offices implement a policy to address patient billing. Follow this policy consistently for all patients.

- ✔ **Document, document, document.** Good documentation practices provide a paper trail that verifies your consistency. Most providers, for example, follow the "three billing cycle statements" rule: They bill patients at least three times before forgiving an outstanding balance. You should document each patient statement in the patient record along with any conversations with the patient or payer.

- ✔ **Know what the contract says.** Payer contracts generally indicate how patient balances are to be handled. Medicare, for example, requires a collection effort for all Medicare patient balances, regardless of the amount. Others usually have similar expectations. If the provider fails to make collection efforts for patient balances, the insurance company may view this as breach of contract and terminate the agreement or deny renegotiation.

✓ **Be aware of the False Claims Act, which makes defrauding government programs a crime.** You can run afoul of this act if you knowingly submit a false claim, cause a false claim to be submitted, or create a false record that results in a fraudulent claim. Billing 30 claims for a day that only shows 20 patients, for example, is a violation of the Act. (Refer to the earlier section "Surviving a sticky situation" for advice on how to deal with employers who try to pressure you into doing things that are unethical or illegal.)

✓ **Know the boundaries of your claim.** You can't ask for money that isn't coded. Pretty simple. Knowing what procedure you can code on any given claim is a vital part of doing your job ethically and accurately. You can find this information in the payer contracts, in the CPT book, and in other coding resources, such as professional publications. You can also ask more experienced coders in your office. (Refer to Chapters 11 through 13 for detailed information on preparing and submitting a claim.)

The cardinal rule of ethical coding is "When in doubt, ask." If you find any ambiguity in the patient record, query the provider to get clarification. As I say throughout this book, any claim must be fully supported by the record.

## Avoiding accusations of fraudulent billing

Attempting to collect balances less than $25 can become costly, so having a write-off policy can save a practice both time and money. In your collection efforts, focus on larger outstanding balances. When balances are forgiven, note the account and, if the patient tries to return, collect all outstanding debts and copays prior to another encounter.

Keep in mind, however, that the only condition under which the provider can't collect an outstanding debt from a patient is if the provider has sent the patient an IRS form 1099 to patients whose debts were forgiven. This form is used to report income on which taxes were not collected. (The 1099 obligates the patient to report the non-paid debt as income, because he or she received something of value and didn't pay for it.)

Providers who routinely forgive patient debt run the risk of prosecution under anti-kickback statutes and possibly the False Claims Act. The reasoning is that, by not collecting co-insurance amounts from patients, providers are billing Medicare for excessive charges. Say Medicare pays $80 of a $100 bill, with the expectation that the patient will pay the remaining $20. By not going after the

$20 patient contribution, the provider is essentially saying that he really only expected to receive $80, not the $100 he actually billed. And if he was expecting only $80 for the service, he shouldn't have billed $100.

To avoid accusations of fraudulent billing, do the following:

- ✔ Consistently apply the office hardship policy to all patients.

- ✔ Keep proof of financial hardship, which should consist of an application for financial assistance that documents the patient's financial stability. Also document all attempts to collect patient debts.

- ✔ Verify the wording in payer contracts with regard to patient balances.

Bottom line: You can forgive patients — but not too much!

# Part VI
# The Part of Tens

## The 5th Wave
By Rich Tennant

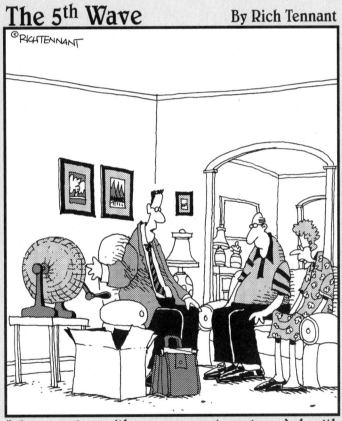

"You can stay with your current employer's health care plan, opt for Medicare Part D, or randomly pick 20 generic drugs from our Rotating Cage of Prescription Drug Coverage Plan."

## In this part . . .

Who loves a list? Well, I do. And I hope you do, too, because I've come up with three useful lists to help you navigate the wide world of medical billing and coding. In the first chapter, I share ten common mistakes to avoid to keep your nose, and your coding, clean. Then I list the top ten need-to-know acronyms you'll hear, see, or use every day. In the last chapter in this part, I share sage advice from medical billing and coding professionals.

# Chapter 19

# Ten Common Billing and Coding Mistakes and How to Avoid Them

## In This Chapter

▶ Avoiding issues with your coding

▶ Protecting your patients and provider

▶ Maintaining your integrity

*R*epeat after me: Ethical violations are bad. As a coder, you must consistently do the right thing at work, especially related to providers, payers, and patients. By virtue of your position, you are privy to sensitive information and have an impact on the financial well-being of all the people who rely on you to do your job. In this chapter, I outline the most egregious of the ethical and legal violations that can land you in hot water if you ever stray from the straight and narrow.

## Being Dishonest

Certified medical coders are trained to abstract billable procedures from the medical record. A true-blue coder respects the rules of coding. The biggest rule is that all the procedures you submit must be documented in the record, not just mentioned in the heading. Therefore, resist the temptation to submit codes that are only implied or that are not documented by medical necessity. Don't unbundle codes for the sake of additional reimbursement and don't choose a procedural code that is "like" the actual service performed. Code honestly, code accurately, and you'll do just fine.

## Shifting the Blame

You have nothing to gain by shifting the blame of inaccurate coding on to others. If you work in an environment with a department for each step of the coding cycle, ask for clarification as to how much leeway you have to facilitate. If you notice that claims are not being submitted in a timely manner, for example, and nothing in the documentation explains the reason for the delay, bring the matter to the attention of the appropriate party. If the entire revenue cycle is your job, then take responsibility to ensure that the claims are moving as they should through the cycle. To maintain your integrity and the respect of your superiors and co-workers, be a team player and stay focused on the bottom line: revenue for your provider or client.

# Billing More Than Is Documented

Physicians often dictate every step of a procedure, but that does not mean that each step is actually billable. To be eligible for separate reimbursement, the procedure must have required additional work and skill by the physician. Stick to the provider's documentation to bill exactly what you need to, no more and no less. If the documentation is ambiguous, take the time to clarify what occurred with the physician. Chapter 12 tells you how to conduct a physician query.

# Unbundling Incorrectly

Codes that are bundled are considered incidental to another billable procedure. For example, a surgeon must make an incision before a surgery can be performed. The incision is incidental, and the surgeon must then close the incision. Again, a normal closure is incidental because it is necessary to complete the primary procedure. The physician usually fully documents the approach (the incision) and the closure, but that doesn't mean that you should bill for them. Similarly, a procedure that is a result of the surgeon "being in the area anyway" is not necessarily billable. The key is to know which procedures are bundled and which ones aren't. You can find this information by checking NCCI edits. If the procedures are considered incidental, they will be included in the bundling edits. Chapters 4 and 12 have the details of bundling.

# Ignoring an Error

Occasionally the documentation has an error. Perhaps it's a transcription error or an omission by the provider. Either way, as the biller/coder, you're responsible for bringing the error to the attention of the physician and making sure that it is corrected. Sometimes resolving the error is as simple as correcting a patient name or a spelling error. Other times, the error may be in the coding — you (or someone else) abstracted the wrong code, for example.

In all cases, after you find and correct the error, you must submit the corrected claim. Failure to do so can result in the provider receiving an undeserved payment or being underpaid. Bottom line: Find the problem and follow up on it immediately to avoid bigger problems later. Go to Chapter 18 for details on what to do when you make an error on your claims.

# Mishandling an Overpayment

Occasionally, a payer fails to process a claim correctly, either paying too much or too little. If a claim has been underpaid, the provider is quick to ask that the error be rectified. When a claim has been overpaid, the same policy should be implemented. If a payer has failed to follow the contract and allowed more than the contract obligates, the provider should notify the payer and prepare to return the erroneous payment. Doing so reinforces your integrity with the payer and also averts potential interest payments that may be obligated when the payer finds the error and asks for reimbursement. For information on how to deal with under- and overpayments and other reimbursement problems, head to Chapter 14.

# Failing to Protect Patients from Out-of-Network Penalties

Most patients are not experts on insurance plans or the medical claim processes. If a provider treats patients out-of-network, the patient usually faces penalties in the form of high deductibles or higher co-insurance liability. Some plans don't cover out-of-network services at all, and the patient is responsible for the entire costs.

To protect patients from this scenario, providers should have office policies that define how out-of-network patients are to be billed. In addition, and whenever possible, you should verify patient benefits prior to any encounter and explain to the patient the provider's expectations regarding to copayments, deductibles, and co-insurance responsibilities. (You can generally find liability information on the patient's insurance card.) For a quick refresher on the different kinds of insurance plans, head to Chapter 6.

# Failing to Verify Prior Authorization

Before they can be performed, some procedures require that the provider receive prior authorization, which is permission from the payer for the patient to be treated. Failure to obtain necessary authorizations or referrals (when a primary care physician sends a patient to another provider for treatment or tests) may result in the claim being denied. Depending upon the provisions of the patient's plan, liability for billed charges then fall on either the provider or the patient.

For this reason, checking whether planned procedures need prior authorization is a vital part of ensuring that the provider adheres to the contract he has with a payer and receives the negotiated reimbursement for the service he provides. Always ask the physician to note any and all procedures that may be performed and check for authorization requirements for each one. Obtaining an authorization that is not needed is better than finding out after the claim is submitted that one was required. For more on referrals and prior authorizations, head to Chapter 11.

# Breaking Patient Confidentiality

As the coder, you have access to both the patient's clinical information and his or her personal demographic information, such as Social Security number, date of birth, address, and so on. It goes without saying that you need to guard this information as you would your own, not only because of the threat of identity theft but also because of ramifications of violating the Health Insurance Portability and Accountability Act (HIPAA). HIPAA governs to whom, under what circumstances, and what kind of information you can share about a patient, and violators may be subject to steep fines and the possibility of imprisonment. For more information about HIPAA and strategies for protecting patient confidentiality, go to Chapter 4.

# Following the Lead of an Unscrupulous Manager

Most coding managers know about and adhere to correct coding processes and expect you to follow those processes as well. Unfortunately, you may encounter an manager who is less aware of correct coding rules or who, if cognizant of the rules, tends to bend or overlook them. These coding managers may see modifiers as a tool to increase reimbursement rather than a tool to increase specificity when reporting services, for example, and may challenge the coding of claims when reimbursement is low.

If your manager or other superior encourages you to code out of bounds, don't acquiesce. Instead, do what you think is right and report the incident to an office leader who can follow up on the matter. You may get on the shady manager's bad side, but you'll be able to sleep much better at night! Chapter 18 offers strategies you can use when you're under pressure to code in questionable or unethical ways.

# Chapter 20

# Ten Acronyms to Burn into Your Brain

*In This Chapter*

▶ Familiarizing yourself with industry lingo

▶ Memorizing the big government names to know

*T*he world of medical billing and coding is like one big bowl of alphabet soup. Just about any term that comes up in your daily dealings has a corresponding acronym. Every office becomes familiar with the abbreviations specific to that particular practice, but some acronyms are known industry wide and are familiar to everyone who works in the healthcare industry. In this chapter, I explain a few more of the most common abbreviations and acronyms that all medical offices use.

Some states regulate the clinical abbreviations and acronyms used in medical records. These state regulations usually require that each abbreviation has only one meaning and that that meaning is documented on a list available to all clinical staff. For administrative staff, however, the acronyms and abbreviations aren't usually regulated, so you may find even more in-house acronyms floating through the office — which isn't necessarily a bad thing. After all, do you really want to walk around saying, "Health Insurance Portability and Accountability Act" all day when you can just say, "HIPAA"?

## OON: Out-of-Network

Out-of-network (OON) refers to insurance plan benefits. An out-of-network provider is one who does not have a contract with the patient's insurance company and, therefore, is not obligated to accept whatever discounted reimbursement the insurance company was able to negotiate with its in-network providers. Every commercial insurance plan outlines the benefit level for members. Usually when a non-contracted provider treats the patient, the benefits are lower. Your patient may have a fairly inexpensive copay for an in-network provider and a much larger copay for an out-of-network provider. Some carriers may not cover out-of-network providers at all!

# INN: In-network

An in-network (INN) provider is one who has a contract with either the insurance company or the network with whom the payer participates. Patients who go to in-network providers usually have to pay less in co-insurance and deductibles. In addition, INN office visits may require that the patient make a copayment at the time of the visit.

# HMO: Health Maintenance Organization

A health maintenance organization (HMO) is a type of insurance coverage or plan that restricts the patient's options when it comes to receiving treatment from a specialist. With an HMO, patients are assigned to a primary care physician who serves as a gatekeeper for the plan and, when the services of a specialist are necessary, typically sends the patient to other in-network providers. If the patient's primary care physician deems the services of an OON provider necessary, then a referral, a prior authorization, or possibly both are required. Patients with only HMO coverage generally do not receive any benefits when they see an out-of-network provider unless their primary care physician gives a referral when no in-network option is available. Chapter 6 has more on HMOs.

# PPO: Preferred Provider Organization

A preferred provider organization (PPO) is a health insurance coverage plan that allows its members to choose providers, including specialists, that are contracted with the payer's network or insurance company. The patient may choose a primary care provider, but doing so isn't required. If the patient does choose a PCP, referrals aren't required. Go to Chapter 6 for more information about the benefits preferred provider organizations offer.

# POS: Point of Service Health Insurance

The point of service (POS) health insurance option is a kind of hybrid plan between an HMO and a PPO. It offers the low cost of HMOs for patients who choose to see only in-network HMO providers. But it also allows members to see out-of-network providers. Patients who choose the out-of-network option are responsible for higher deductibles and copayments. Chapter 6 has more on POS plans.

# EOB: Explanation of Benefits

An explanation of benefits (EOB) is the document that the insurance company issues in response to a claim submission. The EOB reflects how the claim was processed and shows the billed charges, any reductions applied (either by contract, fee schedule, negotiation, or arbitrarily assigned), the allowed amount, and, finally, any remaining patient liability. Patients are billed as indicated by the EOB, meaning that providers can't bill them any additional amount to make up for any discounts applied to the claim. Chapter 13 has info on the EOB and what you, as a biller/coder, need to do with it.

# WC: Workers' Compensation

Workers' Compensation (WC) is insurance that covers employees injured at work. Each Workers' Compensation carrier has filing guidelines, and you want to make sure you know what those requirements are. In addition, Workers' Comp claims are always specific to the body part and condition to be treated; before you file a Worker's' Comp claim, you must verify that the injury and body part treated correspond with the treatment as approved by Worker's Comp.

Some states have fee schedules or payment legislation that must be followed by carriers and accepted by providers. Otherwise, carriers usually seek PPO networks (sometimes silent) to price their claims. Chapter 6 and 16 have more information on Workers' Comp claims and how to deal with them.

# EDI: Electronic Data Interchange

The electronic data interchange (EDI) is the system through which you can electronically transfer medical claims from the provider to the payer. The transfer may route directly from the provider to the payer, or it may go from the provider to a clearinghouse that then sends it on to the payer. EDI allows information to be transmitted in a secure method that protects patient demographic and clinical information. Because EDI reduces the need for paper, it's faster and, therefore, more productive.

# HIPAA: Health Insurance Portability and Accountability Act

The Health Insurance Portability and Accountability Act (HIPAA) was approved by Congress to protect the privacy of patients and insure that patients have access to their medical files. All patients must sign a notice stating that the provider made them aware of their rights, and all employees must sign a confidentiality agreement that states they understand the need to protect patient confidentiality and the penalties involved if they violate HIPAA.

In addition, HIPAA requires patients to identify others (such as a spouse or parent) who can have access to their healthcare information. Under HIPAA, any conversation between a physician and patient is confidential, and information regarding that interaction cannot be left in a voice mail or on an answering machine unless specifically instructed to do so by the patient in writing.

# CMS: Centers for Medicare & Medicaid Services

The Centers for Medicare & Medicaid Services (CMS) is a division of the United States Department of Health & Human Services. CMS administers Medicare, Medicaid, and the Children's Health Insurance Program — programs that serve the most vulnerable segments of the population. In addition to serving these populations, CMS also sets the standard for healthcare, and many commercial payers follow CMS payment guidelines. You can read more about CMS's Medicare and Medicaid programs in Chapters 6 and 17.

# Chapter 21

# Ten Tips from Billing and Coding Pros

*Y*ou've now arrived at the unsolicited advice portion of the book. Usually, that sort of advice is unwelcome, like when your in-laws offer child-rearing advice without asking. But I'm betting you'll find this particular brand of off-the-cuff advice helpful because it comes from seasoned professionals who have walked the same path you're embarking on right now. Think of the pointers in this chapter as your own little coffee klatch, minus the coffee. Here I give you ten tips that will help keep you sane when you're knee-deep in coding.

## Demand Proper Documentation

The revenue cycle begins when the patient completes the demographic form prior to admission and the provider verifies the patient's coverage. The cycle continues when the physician completes his or her documentation of the patient encounter. Your job ultimately depends on all involved parties recording the right kind of info at the right time. This preparation, if done correctly, sets the stage for correct claims processing and payment. To get the information you need, you must make sure that everyone involved is aware of the necessary documentation and works as a team to achieve that goal.

# Verify Patient Benefits

When it comes to paying medical bills (the payers and patients) or receiving reimbursement (the providers), you don't want any surprises. To avoid unpleasant "Gotcha!" moments, call the payer to check for remaining deductibles, co-insurance responsibilities, and any applicable copayments, and collect them prior to admission from the patient. Also verify the need for a prior authorization for any planned procedures. Your goal should be to collect all this information before the patient even walks through the door of the provider's office.

# Get Vital Patient Info at Check-in

Collect patient demographics (name, address, date of birth, phone number, marital status, employer, Social Security number, and so on), and get a copy of the insurance card upon patient arrival. You need this information when the time comes to code and submit the claim.

Also verify patient identification. Institute a policy, if your office doesn't have one already, that all patients must present a government-issued form of ID upon arrival; then make a copy of that ID and place in the record. Don't be left holding the bag just because you forgot to ask for a photo ID.

# Review the Documentation ASAP

As a biller/coder, you rely on the documentation. It has the physician's notes regarding diagnosis and treatment, as well as the demographic information you need. Although you technically have a few days before you must code and send the claim off, don't delay. Your goal should be to have the claim out the door within 72 hours. Review the medical documentation as soon as possible after the encounter or procedure to see whether it is as complete as you need it to be. And if you find any omissions or ambiguities to clarify, query the physician as soon as possible.

# Set Up a System to Ensure Accuracy

From coding to reimbursement, the biller/coder has to perform several tasks: abstracting all billable codes and supporting diagnosis codes from the record; entering the claim into the billing software in preparation for claim submission and then submitting it; checking the clearinghouse submission reports; and following up on any problems or denials. To do this job well, you must be both accurate and efficient.

Depending upon the office structure, you need time management skills to get everything done on time. Your primary job is to get the claim to the payer and then to follow up to make sure the claim was received and is being processed. Your back-end job is to appeal claims that have not paid correctly. If coding and billing in the morning and spending afternoons doing follow up is a reasonable schedule for you, then plan accordingly.

# Play Nice with Others

On its way to generating reimbursement, your claim will go either directly to the payer or to a clearinghouse first and then to the payer. In either place, it can get hung up. If claims are rejecting at the clearinghouse, work with the people there to identify the underlying reason.

If the payer is unable to accept your electronic claims (which may happen when the payer implements a new processing system or transitions from one platform to another), send your claims on paper until the problem is resolved. If your billing software is the problem (for example, claim forms not populating correctly), work with the software vendor to resolve the issue.

Regardless of what the problem ends up being — or where it occurs — the best way to quickly resolve an issue is to make the person you're talking to feel like you and she are a team working on the problem together. Remember: Be friendly, and you will yield results in the process!

# Follow Up on Accounts Receivable Daily

Putting claims through the process may be the main focus of your job, but making sure the money comes through is just as important. Set time aside each day to review the accounts receivable reports (making sure that you're always working with the latest report). Be sure to pay attention to whether the claims have been received; then watch the accounts receivable aging reports (which are generated by your billing software and show all the outstanding claims and the dollar amounts associated with each) to monitor all outstanding accounts. If you see that some are stalled, get on the horn with the payer to resolve the issue.

# Be a Bulldog on the Phone

Persistence pays off. So does being clear on what you need and expect. So for every claim over 60 days old, call the payer. Verify that the claim is in process and make note of the claim number and when payment can be expected. If the representative tells you that the payment has been issued, get the date, check number, and the amount of the check (note whether it was it a bulk check or single check). You can also verify the address the check was sent to and ask whether it has presented for payment or cashed.

# Know Your Payer Contracts by Heart

The more familiar you are with all payer contracts, the more quickly and accurately you can process claims. Payer contracts stipulate things like what procedures are covered and whether prior authorization or referrals are needed. They also outline billing requirements, such as how long you have to submit the claim (called timely filing), how long the payer has to make payment before interest is earned, and other payer specific quirks, such as revenue code requirements or value codes that are expected.

As you become an expert on the details of the payer contracts, be sure to note any updates and changes (policies and benefit levels change regularly). Most payers post policy revisions and additions on their websites, but with regard to individual contracts, you need to know where your employer keeps these documents. They may be on a company server, kept in the manager's drawer, or held in a binder on your desk.

# Create a File System That Lets You Find What You Need

If you or anybody else ever has a question about the status of a claim, the last thing you want to have to do is root around your office space looking for the relevant documentation. By creating a system that tells you instantly when things are received and where you can find them, you can more easily keep track of your claims and retrieve the necessary info whenever you need to.

For example, use a date stamp to document when you receive payments and explanation of benefits (EOBs) and keep a daily file of all received payments and non-payment claim documents. For most small- to intermediate-sized offices, this can be as simple as keeping each day's EOBs in a file folder. Then for each document that is claim related, note the account, what was received, the date it was received, and how it relates to the account. Link the payment for each claim to the date the EOB was received and note each account of non-payment documents, including when they were received. That way if you need to refer to one of these documents, you know where to find it.

# Make Payers Show You the Money!

Your primary objective as a biller and coder is to make sure that your employer is reimbursed appropriately for the services he provides. That means you can't let him be underpaid. To guard against the provider being underpaid, make sure you follow up and appeal any claim that does not pay as expected. If your provider has a contract with a payer and the claim didn't pay according to the contract, you can base your argument solely on the contract. If no contract exists between the provider and payer, call the payer and ask what method was used to price the claim. Claims that were paid "usual and customary" should be challenged. If a silent PPO was accessed (you can find out more about those in Chapter 16), ask for the contract to be identified and then notify the network in writing that you wish to terminate the relationship.

# Glossary

**AAPC (formerly the American Academy of Professional Coders).** The nation's largest training and credentialing organization for medical coders.

**accounts receivable (AR):** The industry name for outstanding payments. For most companies, 90 days in AR is acceptable, although most contracts contain language that obligates payment within a certain time.

**acute injury:** Damage to the body incurred by accident.

**adjudication:** Payment obligation according to the patient's insurance benefits with regard to a claim.

**advanced beneficiary notice (ABN):** A notice the provider may ask a Medicare beneficiary to sign for a service or item that will probably not be covered. By signing an ABN, the patient agrees to be financially responsible in the event that Medicare denies payment. If the patient is not notified or doesn't sign the notice before services are rendered, then he or she does not have to pay for it.

**American Health Information Management Association (AHIMA):** The official association of health information management professionals.

**anatomy:** The study of the human body structure.

**arthroscopic surgery:** A surgical technique, using tiny cameras, employed by orthopedic surgeons, that allows them to visualize, diagnose, and possibly treat injury or disease inside a joint.

**body system:** A group of organs that performs a specific task.

**bundling:** The grouping together of one or more CPT codes that are considered incidental or inclusive to another and that should not be reimbursed individually. For these additional codes to be considered for separate payment, the physician must describe the extra work performed, including the extra time involved and why it was necessary.

**Centers for Medicare & Medicaid Services (CMS):** A branch of the United States Department of Health & Human Services that administers Medicare and Medicaid.

**Certified Coding Associate (CCA):** An AHIMA certification that shows the recipient has demonstrated the ability to abstract the correct procedural and diagnosis codes in hospitals and physician practices.

**Certified Coding Specialist (CCS):** An AHIMA certification that indicates competency in hospital coding and requires a higher level of expertise in diagnosis and procedural coding. CCS-certified coders also possess a strong knowledge of medical terminology and human anatomy.

**Certified Professional Coder (CPC):** AAPC certification that indicates proficiency in reading medical charts and abstracting the correct diagnosis codes, procedural codes, and supply codes. CPC-certified coders also have at least two years of experience in the coding profession.

**Certified Professional Coder Apprentice (CPC-A):** The initial AAPC certification indicating that the coder is an apprentice. After completing a 2-year apprenticeship in coding or billing in a medical office, the CPC-A coder can request that the *A* be removed.

**chronic injury:** Damage that is a result of overuse or aging.

**claims matching:** The process that occurs when specific services are performed by several providers who submit claims for the same patient.

**claims processing:** The overall work of receiving a claim from the provider and determining eligibility for payment.

**claims scrubbing:** The process by which the editing system checks the claim for errors and verifies that it is compatible with the payer software before sending the claim to the payer.

**claims submission:** The process of sending to the payer the procedural codes that represent the work performed by the healthcare provider.

**commercial insurance carrier:** The company that writes the reimbursement check to the provider.

**compliance:** When an office or individual has set up a program to run the practice under the regulations set forth by the United States Office of Inspector General (OIG).

**consultation:** A visit with a physician specialist that has specific requirements that must be met (the visit must be requested from an authorized source, must be accompanied by an opinion from your provider, and must include a response to the requesting physician) before the claim can be billed.

**contract payers:** Payers with whom a provider has a contract or payers that are part of a network with whom the provider has a contract.

**contracted carve-out:** A special clause in the contract that allows certain procedures to be reimbursed at a different rate from the rate specified by the procedural code.

**CPT (current procedural terminology) books:** The books published annually by the American Medical Association (AMA) that contain all procedural codes billed. The codes are based on the procedures defined by the AMA.

**critical care codes:** Time-based codes used when a patient is critically ill and that support a high level of reimbursement. Per CPT guidelines, these codes include specific care that must be completed in order to bill.

**definitive diagnosis:** A diagnosis made after the body cavity becomes visible (that is, after the surgeon has either opened up the patient or inserted a scope to see the patient's inner workings).

**Department of Health & Human Services (HHS):** The primary U.S. government agency responsible for protecting the health of Americans. Medicare and Medicaid, part of the Centers for Medicare & Medicaid Services, are two of this agency's programs.

**diagnosis terms:** Terms that determine medical necessity as defined by the payers.

**diagnosis-related groups (DRGs):** The way in which an admitting diagnosis is linked to the severity of the patient's illness. Hospitals are reimbursed based on DRGs.

**diagnostic laparoscopy:** A diagnostic procedure using a scope.

**disease process:** A deviation of the normal structure or function of a body part that is represented by symptoms.

**EDI (Electronic Data Interchange):** The electronic systems that carry claims to a central clearinghouse for distribution to individual carriers.

**electronic data interchange number (EDI):** An electronic number that serves as the payer's "address" or identifier. This number tells the clearinghouse which payer to send the claim to.

**electronic health record (EHR):** An electronic record of a patient's health history. EHRs are intended to do away with paper charts, thus making protecting and sharing health information easier.

**evaluation and management (E&M) codes:** The codes representing non-invasive physician services that are used for every office visit or encounter a physician has with a patient. Typically these encounters involve taking a history, an examination, and decision making on the part of the provider. These are the most commonly billed codes.

**evaluation and management encounter:** A doctor's visit, also known as an E&M visit. E&M visits may take place in a physician's office, nursing home, hospital, emergency room, or clinic.

**fibrosis:** A condition resulting from excess fibrous connective tissue that is trying to heal itself.

**first-level appeal:** A friendly reminder to a payer that the contract was not followed or that a discount was applied without a contract.

**Health Insurance Portability and Accountability Act (HIPAA):** The law, sometimes called the Privacy rule, outlining how certain entities like health plans or clearinghouses can use or disclose personal health information. Under HIPAA, patients must be allowed access to their medical records.

**Health Maintenance Organization (HMO):** Health management plan that requires the patient to use a primary care physician who acts as a gatekeeper to other health services. In HMOs, patients much seek treatment from the primary physician first, who, if she feels the situation warrants it, can refer the patient to a specialist within the network.

**Healthcare Common Procedure Coding System (HCPCS) book:** Code books used for various services, drugs, and other medical equipment not found in the CPT book.

**Healthcare Financing Administration (HCFA) form:** The paper form, also known as the CMS-1500 form, that physicians and clinical practitioners use to submit claims for professional services.

**healthcare spending account (HSA):** A spending account funded pre-tax by the insured party.

**healthcare reimbursement account (HRA):** An account funded by the employer that reimburses patients for money spent on out-of-pocket health-care costs.

**illness:** A feeling or condition of not being healthy.

**implied procedure:** A procedure that is listed in the heading of a record but is not documented in the body of the record.

**inpatient:** A person who has been officially admitted to the hospital under a physician's order. The patient remains an inpatient until the day before the day of discharge.

**intermediary:** The network that priced the claim for the payer.

**laparoscopy:** A procedure in which the physician views or performs surgery in the abdominal cavity via a tiny camera.

**manual processing:** The act of processing claims that must be reviewed by a human, not just a computer system.

**Medicaid:** The federal program created by the 1965 Social Security Act that helps low-income people pay for part or all of their medical bills. The U.S. Department of Health & Human Services regulates the Medicaid program, but each state is responsible for its own program administration. These programs are completely voluntary, but each state has some form of Medicaid program available to eligible residents.

**medical biller:** The person responsible for correctly billing insurance companies and patients.

**medical coder:** The person responsible for deciphering the documentation and determining the appropriate CPT and diagnosis code(s) that represent the services provided.

**medical necessity:** The reason for the visit or surgery that defines the disease process or injury.

**medical terminology:** Terms that describe illness, injury, conditions, and procedures.

**Medicare:** The federal health insurance program for people 65 years or older, under age 65 with certain disabilities, and any age with end-stage renal disease or Lou Gehrig's disease. Medicare has four parts: Part A (hospital insurance), Part B (medical insurance), Part C (known as Medicare Advantage Plans), and Part D (prescription drug coverage).

**Medicare Administrative Contractor (MAC):** The area contractor with the fiduciary contract with CMS to administer payments and denials to providers for Medicare Part A and Medicare Part B claims. MACs encompass several states, and their areas are listed on the CMS website.

**Medicare Appeals Council (MAC):** Part of the Departmental Appeals Board of the U.S. Department of Health & Human Services that provides the final administrative review of claims filed by beneficiaries or healthcare providers and suppliers relating to Medicare entitlements, coverage, and payment.

**missing procedure:** A procedure for which a diagnosis is listed but no treatment is noted.

**modifiers:** Alphanumeric symbols used to indicate that the published description of a service or supply has been altered.

**multiple procedure discount:** The discount applied to the second, third, or any additional procedures when multiple procedures are paid.

**multiple procedure reduction (MPD):** A pay rate scale in which the first procedure is paid at 100 percent of contractual allowance, while the second may be paid at a reduced rate (often 50 percent), and the third at whatever percentage is deemed appropriate per the contract.

**mutually exclusive procedure:** A procedure that can't be performed or coded in combination with another. An example would be coding for a fracture repair on the left forearm and then coding for an amputation of the left forearm.

**National Correct Coding Initiative (NCCI) edits:** Edits established by CMS to help insure correct coding and eliminate inappropriate coding and reporting. NCCI edits indicate which procedures are incidental to (or included with) another specific CPT code.

**National Provider Identifier (NPI):** A unique identification number assigned to covered healthcare providers and that must be used by health plans and healthcare clearinghouses. HIPAA laws require the use of this number.

**network:** Essentially a middleman that functions as an agent for commercial payers. Payers may participate with a network that contracts healthcare providers, and the network will price the claims for the payer according to the contract.

**non-contracted payers:** Payers with whom the provider does not have a contract. Payment for these claims is considered out-of-network and needs to be carefully investigated prior to any patient encounter.

**Office of Inspector General (OIG):** The federal office that provides oversight for the U.S. Department of Health & Human Services and programs under other HHS institutions, including the Centers for Disease Control and Prevention, the National Institutes of Health, and the Food and Drug Administration.

**Office of Medicare Hearings and Appeals (OMHA):** The federal office, created by the Medicare Modernization Act of 2003, whose purpose is to streamline and make the appeals process more efficient. OMHA is responsible for the level-three Medicare appeals process.

**open procedure:** A procedure in which a patient's body is cut open.

**open surgery:** The term used to refer to traditional procedures involving an incision made by surgeon.

**operative report:** The information that the physician dictates, which is then transcribed into a written document that details exactly what was done during the surgery.

**outpatient:** A patient who comes to a hospital or other facility but has not been admitted as a patient, even if spending the night. Outpatients may come through the emergency room or may be undergoing tests or minor surgery.

**payer:** The entity that reimburses the provider for services. Insurance companies, government programs like Medicare and Medicaid, and third-party administrators are all payers in the healthcare industry.

**payment floor:** A set length of time the payer has to complete and process claims.

**physician query:** The process of asking a physician for clarification about documentation.

**portal:** An incision made either for visualization or used to insert instruments or a camera.

**preauthorization:** The process of getting an agreement from the payer to cover specific services before the service is performed; also known as *prior authorization*.

**Preferred Provider Organization (PPO):** Health management plan that allows patients to visit any providers contracted with their insurance companies. If the patient visits a non-contracted provider, the claim is considered out-of-network.

**prefix:** The beginning segment of the word. In medical terminology, the prefix is the first indication of the area where the procedures may be located.

**preoperative diagnosis:** A diagnosis made prior to an operation, based on test findings and examination.

**Professional Medical Coding Curriculum (PMCC) instructor:** The AAPC certification indicating that an individual has received additional instruction above and beyond a coding certification and has passed the certification tests and is, therefore, qualified to teach coding courses.

**relative value unit (RVU):** A monetary value assigned to every CPT code that represents the amount of work necessary to perform the procedure.

**retired modifiers:** Modifiers that were removed from the Medicare list and are no longer valid for Medicare. Commercial payers that use older processing software may still use retired modifiers.

**revenue cycle:** The process, from beginning to end, of translating the work performed by the doctor and his staff into payment. The cycle begins with the appointment and ends with payment from the carrier or patient.

**scope families:** Procedures that go together. This designation is used when performing an additional, related procedure that does not require additional time or skill by the surgeon and, therefore, is not eligible for additional reimbursement.

**scope procedure:** A procedure in which a minimally invasive scope (or tiny camera) is used to perform a procedure inside the body.

**second-level appeal:** A more formal appeal, sent after a first-level appeal has failed to resolve an issue. Any information not previously given should be submitted with this appeal.

**suffix:** The ending section of the word that, in medical terminology, describes the condition of the area being treated or action that was taken.

**super-bill:** A billing form created specifically for an individual office or provider that is generally pre-populated with the patient's information and contains the most common diagnosis and procedural codes used by the office.

**surgical field:** The area being operated on.

**tax ID number:** An identifying number for a business. (Think of it as a business's Social Security number.)

**third-party administrator (TPA):** Intermediaries who either operate as a network or access networks to price claims. TPAs often handle claims processing for employers who self-insure their employees rather than use a traditional group health plans.

**transmission format:** Uniform format in which claim information is sent and received. The template indicates the service received, the reason for the service, the cost of the service, and information identifying the patient and the provider.

**Tricare:** The healthcare system, funded by the U.S. Department of Defense, that active and retired military and their dependents use.

**unbundling:** Coding procedure in which the coder includes additional codes on the claim that represent procedures that were incidental to the primary procedure.

**underwriting:** When a commercial carrier uses the health history and age of employees to price healthcare policies for small companies providing healthcare for their employees. The company then accepts liability for costs incurred under the policy.

**Uniform Bill 04 (UB-04) form:** The claim form used by facilities, rather than physicians, for their health insurance billing. The UB-O4 form is also called the CMS-1450.

**up-coding:** Billing for a higher level of service than was performed. Up-coding may be considered fraud if it's done over time with intention.

**write-off:** The part of the claim not paid by the payer or the patient and that is forgiven. A write-off can also be referred to as a discount.

# Index

## • F •

hospital, working environment, 33–34
hospital visit, 74–76
HRA (healthcare reimbursement account), 82, 297
HSA (healthcare spending account), 48, 82, 296
human anatomy. *See* body systems
*hyper-* prefix, 62
hypertension, 64
*hypo-* prefix, 62
hypotension, 64
hypothalamus, 134
*hyster-* prefix, 62

## • I •

*-ia* suffix, 63
ICD (International Classification of Diseases), 17–18, 225–226
ICD-9 (ICD, 9th edition)
  compared to ICD-10, 226–227
  linking CPT codes to, 180
  moving to ICD-10 from, 17–18, 227, 230–233
  symbols in, 53
  using in certification exam, 142–143
ICD-10 (ICD, 10th edition)
  compared to ICD-9, 226–227
  5010 transmission platform for, 228–230
  moving to, from ICD-9, 17–18, 227, 230–233
  symbols in, 53
ICD-11 (ICD, 11th edition), 233–234
ICD-CM (ICD, clinical modification), 225
ICD-PCS (ICD, procedure coding system), 225
icons used in this book, 5
identification of patient, 162
illness, 59–60, 297
implied procedure, 297
incidental procedures, 51, 70
independent audits, 268
individual payer. *See* commercial insurance carrier
injuries
  acute, 293
  chronic, 294
  described, 60–61
INN (in-network) provider, 284

inpatient, 297
inpatient codes, 75
insurance. *See* commercial insurance carrier; government payers
insurance benefits, verifying, 162, 203–204, 247–248, 256–257, 288
insurance commissioner, 176
insurance company. *See* commercial insurance carrier
integumentary system, 59, 134
*inter-* prefix, 62
interactive voice response system (IVR) system, 87, 255
intermediary, 297
internal audits, 54
internal medicine, specialty certification for, 150
International Classification of Diseases (ICD), 17–18, 225–226
internships, 40, 120
interventional radiology, specialty certification for, 150
intestine, 62, 134
*intra-* prefix, 62
involuntary muscles, 137
IRS 1099 form, 274
*-itis* suffix, 63
IVR (interactive voice response) system, 87, 255

## • J •

jobs. *See also* claims processor; medical biller; medical coder
  certification for. *See* certification
  first job, finding, 36
  goals for, 14–15, 112–113
  job market, researching, 105
  requirements for, 15, 111–114
  types of, choosing, 13–15, 24, 28–30
  working environment of. *See* working environment
joints, 62, 136
*Journal of AHIMA* (publication), 269